Springer Series: THE TEACHING OF NURSING

Series Editor: Diane McGivern, RN, PhD, FAAN

Carol Noll Hoskins, PhD, RN, FAAN, Professor of Nursing at New York University, served as Director of the Program in Research and Theory Development in Nursing Science (1985–1990). Her research is on adjustment of the family to illness, repeated measures designs, and psychometrics. She is the author of two measures of interactive behaviors in the partner relationship, *The Partner Relationship Inventory* and *The Dominance-Accommodation Scale.*

Professor Hoskins was principal investigator for a longitudinal study of psychosocial adjustment of women with breast cancer and their partners (1990–1996). She is primary author on numerous publications in which the findings are presented. The findings were used to develop a four-part instructional videotape series, *Journey to Recovery: For Women with Breast Cancer and their Partners.* The phase-specific content is applicable to the diagnostic, postsurgical, adjuvant therapy, and ongoing recovery periods.

As an exchange professor in India, visiting scholar in both Finland and Thailand, and Fulbright scholar in Greece, Professor Hoskins has taught clinical research methods, theory development, principles of measurement, and psychosocial nursing. Her recent awards include a Senior Fulbright Award, University of Athens, Greece (1995); the Distinguished Alumnus Award, Cornell University—New York Hospital School of Nursing (1995); Professor of the Year, School of Education, New York University (1996); the Joan M. Stout Visiting Scholar, Lienhard School of Nursing, Pace University (1996–1998); and the Honorary Doctorate, University of Athens, Greece (1998).

Developing Research in Nursing and Health

Quantitative and Qualitative Methods

Carol Noll Hoskins
PhD, RN, FAAN

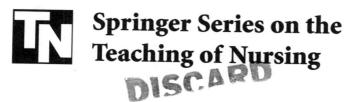

Springer Series on the Teaching of Nursing

Springer Publishing Company, Inc.
536 Broadway
New York, NY 10012-3955

Cover design by Margaret Dunin
Acquisitions Editor: Sheri W. Sussman
Production Editor: T. Orrantia

98 99 00 01 02 / 5 4 3 2 1

Library of Congress Cataloging-in-Publication

Developing research in nursing and health: quantitative and qualitative methods / [edited by] Carol Noll Hoskins.
    p. cm. — (Springer series on the teaching of nursing)
  Includes bibliographical references and index.
  ISBN 0-8261-1185-8 (soft cover)
    1. Nursing—Research—Methodology I. Hoskins, Carol Noll, 1932-. II. Series: Springer series on the teaching of nursing (unnumbered)
    [DNLM: 1. Nursing Research—methods handbooks. 2. Research Design handbooks.
WY 49 G946 1998]
RT81.5.G85 1998
610.73'072—dc21
DNLM/DLC
for Library of Congress   98-10333
                                              CIP

Printed in the United States of America

Contents

Preface

This book was designed to present the basic elements of conducting and understanding nursing research in a quick reference format. The primary motivation for the book came from my many students in the Program in Research and Theory Development at New York University. The first versions of the chapters emerged from the requests of students to have seminars in the doctoral program reinforced by written handouts that were succinct and easy to use. Over the years, the guides were revised and edited and used in other settings, including academic settings in Thailand, India, Finland, and Greece. Although it was originally created for doctoral students, the material can be used by students at the B.S.N. and master's levels, and by practicing nurses.

Chapter 1 provides a review of the basic reasons why nurses need to be involved as consumers or designers of research. It stresses that the challenge of constant evaluation of patient care and the study of how it might be revised in the interest of improving outcomes in patients and families must be a commitment.

In chapter 2, the complexities of identifying and refining a research question are addressed. The research question, whether quantitative or qualitative, provides direction to the entire study, including the design that will be used to seek answers. Although there are various techniques and views on conducting a literature review, the primary sources relevant to nursing with general guides for their use are presented in chapter 3. Most investigators agree that the main aim for a review of the literature should be a comprehensive knowledge of the work that has already been conducted. Accomplishing this objective will enable an investigator to avoid the risk of developing a study, and interpreting the findings, in a relative vacuum.

The next three chapters of the book are focused on the methodological aspects of planning and conducting research. There is much to be learned about research designs, sampling, and data analyses and interpretation. The main points are outlined and can serve as a starting point, while those who seek more information can consult more comprehensive references. The content in the chapters is supplemented by appendixes in which critiquing guides, exemplar studies, and a more detailed discussion of hypothesis testing are provided.

In the last two chapters, the principles of measurement and the process for developing a quantitative measure with alternate forms are addressed. These chapters are included primarily because of nursing investigators' increasing emphasis on the construction of instruments that are sensitive to the behavioral responses that are of particular interest to nurses. Although there has been substantial progress in the endeavor, the standards that have been set by other disciplines in earlier years merit serious consideration. There is a continuing need to develop and evaluate instruments within a sound theoretical context.

In addition to the many responsibilities of their personal lives, nurses are busy professionals. It is hoped that this brief book will prove to be a useful and expeditious guide to those who intend to develop research, collaborate in conducting research, or simply learn about the various parts of the research process.

Acknowledgments

There are a number of colleagues who have made invaluable contributions to this publication. Carla Mariano, RN, EdD, contributed the sections pertaining to qualitative research. As an associate professor in the Division of Nursing at New York University, Dr. Mariano is instrumental in teaching qualitative content and guiding students in the dissertation endeavor. Dr. Mariano has conducted qualitative research in gerontology and interdisciplinarity and has presented her research nationally and internationally. Dr. Mariano's publications include those on the qualitative research process, the case study method, instructional strategies for teaching qualitative research, interdisciplinary collaboration, and aging. She is the recipient of the Distinguished Achievement in Nursing Education Award from Teachers College, Columbia University, and the Rose and George Doval Award for Excellence in Education.

Joseph Giacquinta, EdD, provided the content for the chapter on "Sampling—Basic Issues and Concepts," one of his many areas of expertise in the research process. Dr. Giacquinta is professor of educational sociology in the School of Education at New York University. Part of his role is as coordinator of the School's Interdepartmental Research Studies. He has taught graduate courses on survey research and case study design. He has a long record of quantitative and qualitative research and writing in the field of planned educational change, especially the initiation and implementation of school innovations. He is author of a status-related risk theory of receptivity to change. Among his publications are *Implementing Organizational Innovations* (1971) and *Beyond Technology's Promise* (1993).

Harriet R. Feldman, PhD, RN, FAAN, dean and professor of nursing at the Lienhard School of Nursing at Pace University, contributed the section on the development of vignettes as a measurement technique. She has been an active proponent of research through her service as chairperson of the Council on Nursing Research of the New York State Nurses Association (1992–94) and as chairperson of the statewide Task Force on Nursing Research (1993–94). Her own research and publications are focused on pain perception and management. She is cofounder and coeditor of the journal *Scholarly Inquiry for Nursing Practice*. Dr. Feldman serves as a reviewer for the *Journal of Professional Nursing* and the *Online Journal of Knowledge Synthesis for Nursing* and is a member of the editorial advisory board of the *Journal of the New York State Nurses Association*.

Donald Yucht, recipient of the EdD from New York University, contributed the content on the review of the literature and primary resources for nursing. Dr. Yucht is librarian for technology at New York University's Bobst Library, where his responsibilities include selection of materials for medicine, nursing, food and nutrition, speech language pathology, audiology, and occupational therapy and physical therapy. Formerly, Dr. Yucht served as head of the Instructional Materials Center, head of Special Areas, head of Reader's Session, library coordinator for the Bobst Library, and head of circulation for the General University Library.

CAROL NOLL HOSKINS
New York University

1

Introduction to Research

Increasingly, the research process has been conducted under enormous pressures of time, competition for funds, and other factors that have had a tremendous influence on society in general. Computer technology and databases are intended to make previous studies, including theoretical framework, design, measurement, sample, analyses, and findings, available in the aggregate within moments. Secondary reviews of literature are available for those who decide against primary sources. Although theory development remains an important part of the development and conduct of research, thoughtful attention to the process, as well as other components of the process, becomes more and more problematic.

In chapter 1, the basic reasons for conducting nursing research are reviewed. Although they are not new, they remain sound. Of increasing importance is research on outcomes that are sensitive measures of nursing practice. Further, in the world of managed care, health care system variables as antecedents to outcomes demand increasing attention in nursing research.

In keeping with the pace of modern times, the chapters in this book are primarily in outline form. The reader can, with ease, note the essential points for each topic without the distraction of text. The reader is strongly urged, however, to seek other references when further information is required. A list of some basic research texts is given in the References.

I. INTRODUCTION TO RESEARCH IN NURSING

A. Importance of research to nursing

1. Practice

   a. Understand clients' experiences
   b. Quality of care and outcomes
   c. Cost-effectiveness of care

2. Professionalism

    a.   Scientific base for practice
    b.   Body of knowledge that is distinct from other professions

3. Accountability

    a.   Base decisions and actions in practice, administration, and education on scientifically documented knowledge
    b.   Seek scientific answers to professional issues
    c.   Read the scientific literature for new knowledge and apply to nursing practice, administration, and education

4. Social relevance of nursing

    a.   Nursing, more than ever, is required by consumers and sources of reimbursement to document its role in the delivery of health services

       — Of what benefit is nursing?
       — Can it be documented that nursing care makes a difference?
       — Of what social and practical relevance is nursing?

In summary, most nurses in the United States agree that a large component of nursing practice is—or should be—based on science and that scientific knowledge is developed through research. The research process is a method for posing scientific questions and seeking answers to them. It is a critical function for any profession that claims to base its practice on science.

Without research programs to build its knowledge, a profession is limited to existing knowledge that is often inadequate, or to knowledge developed by other disciplines that may not be appropriate to the problems of the professional practice in question.

B. Kinds of research

1. Basic

    a.   Establish new knowledge or facts
    b.   Develop theories or conceptual frameworks
    c.   Results are not immediately applicable to real-world situations

2. Applied

    a.   Attempts to find solutions to practical problems
    b.   Applies new knowledge relatively soon

II. RELATIONSHIP OF THEORY TO QUANTITATIVE RESEARCH

The theoretical framework within which a given problem is lodged is of crucial importance in every stage of the research. A theory is a systematic explanation of some phenomenon, broader and more complex than a fact. It identifies the variables needed to explain the phenomenon and suggests the nature of the relationships among the variables.

"If a particular problem on which one proposes to do research is not related to an existing theory, does not grow out of an existing theory, is not contained within a newly formed theory, or does not appear capable of altering or confirming a theory, it is most likely irrelevant, useless, and unimportant for consideration as a research problem, especially if [of] an experimental or explanatory nature" (Geitgey & Metz, 1973, pp. 1–5).

A. Theory

    1.   Consists of

        a.   the interrelationships of what is known to be true from research evidence
        b.   what is assumed to be true on the basis of writings by scientists and theoreticians

    2.   Serves to

        a.   explain
        b.   predict
        c.   give direction to research by specifying the variables that need to be measured prior to conducting the research
        d.   provide a framework of variables within which the findings may be compared and integrated with the results of other research

    3.   Assists in selecting the most appropriate variables from which to design the research and guides in their definitions
    4.   Determines the statement and direction of the hypotheses and the subsequent interpretation of findings
    5.   Provides the theoretical basis for linking variables

        a.   The variables may not be arbitrarily linked. They must have empirical or theoretical support for coexistence and testing.
        b.   Logic is used in defining the relationships between variables, e.g., if *A is related to B*, and *B is related to C*, then perhaps *A is related to C*.

III. THE NATURE OF QUALITATIVE RESEARCH

   A. Characteristics

   "The qualitative approach is interactive; context dependent; holistic; flexible, dynamic, and evolving; naturalistic; process oriented; primarily inductive; and descriptive. It has as its foci, perspectives, meanings, uniqueness, and subjective live experiences. Its aim is understanding" (Mariano, 1990, p. 354). Qualitative research methods enable us to explore concepts that we experience in our everyday lives, such as empathy, hope, suffering, caring, fear; to explore these concepts as they are perceived and defined by real people; and to allow people to speak for themselves, thereby emphasizing the human capacity to know (Mariano, 1995).

   1. Use of the natural setting
   2. Emphasis on exploration and discovery versus testing and verifying predetermined hypotheses
   3. Focus on the complexity and wholeness of the phenomenon of human experience—appreciates multiple realities
   4. There is a humanistic orientation
   5. There is direct, close, and prolonged contact with the participants
   6. Attends to temporal, social, and historical contexts
   7. The researcher is the human instrument
   8. The design emerges
   9. Participant observation and in-depth interviewing are frequently used
   10. The study generates an understanding of the human experience often through extensive description or grounded theory

2
The Research Question

The most important initial step in developing research is the identification and phrasing of the research question. This is a process that occurs over time as one reviews the literature and examines studies for questions that have been studied previously. Identifying the constructs, understanding how they have been conceptualized, and evaluating the rationale for linking them are key parts of the endeavor. As studies are located and critiqued, the investigators' phrasing of their own research question is likely to be revised a number of times. If there is little or no work on a particular topic of interest, then the investigator needs to consider approaching the research question from a qualitative perspective.

In chapter 2, the sources and characteristics of quantitative and qualitative research questions are presented. Guides are provided for phrasing each kind of question. In the case of a quantitative question, the kinds of hypotheses and criteria for phrasing them are considered. While the outline format is intended to highlight the key points in a succinct manner, the reader needs to remember that the process requires substantial time, care, and thought that, in the long run, will be worth it.

I.   SOURCES OF RESEARCH QUESTIONS

   A.   Practice
   B.   Nursing theory
   C.   Literature
   D.   Previous research
   E.   Nursing models
   F.   Phenomena inherent in the human condition
   G.   Social concerns

IIa. THE RESEARCH PROBLEM (QUANTITATIVE)

   A.   Consists of *variables* that are

1. constructs or properties studied in research
2. a property that takes on different values (varies)

   a. continuous
   b. dichotomous

3. usually represented by a symbol
4. two major kinds

   a. independent variable

      — presumed "cause" of the dependent variable
      — referred to as X
      — in experimental research, the variable that is manipulated by the experimenter
      — the variable predicted from

   b. dependent variable

      — presumed effect of independent variable
      — referred to as Y
      — the variable predicted to

IIb. THE PROBLEM (QUALITATIVE)

Since the specific problem that actually becomes the focus of the study often *emerges during* the fieldwork, it is likely to be more tentative than in quantitative research.

A. Aim of the study (qualitative)

   1. Consists of

      a. description of the focus of inquiry—what is the phenomenon of interest, what is the event or situation or question to be explored?
      b. context of the phenomenon—the milieu of the phenomenon
      c. context of the researcher

         — researcher's experiences, background, assumptions, precon-ceptions, intuitions, root of interest in the phenomenon
         — researcher's expertise in the method (including preliminary fieldwork)

      d. purpose of the inquiry, e.g., theory building, descriptive base for practice

    e.   succinct overview of the method selected and rationale for why that method is appropriate for this study

    f.   significance of inquiring about this phenomenon

- — Why is it important to study?
- — relevance of the inquiry
- — Why is it necessary to utilize a qualitative design?
- — contribution of the study to understanding, knowledge, practice, and importance to nursing

IIIa. PHRASING THE RESEARCH QUESTION (QUANTITATIVE)

A.   An interrogative sentence that asks, "What relation exists between two or more variables?"

    Ex. Is social support related to patients' and husbands' psychosocial adjustment to breast cancer?

B.   Criteria for research questions

1. Express a relation between two or more variables
2. State clearly and unambiguously in question form
3. Imply possibilities for empirical testing
4. Specify the nature of the population being studied
5. Be introduced early in a research report, with a brief statement of the experiential and scientific background that led to the study

IIIb. PHRASING THE RESEARCH QUESTION (QUALITATIVE)

A.   A question that asks how an individual or group experiences or perceives a particular phenomenon or creates meaning—what is being experienced? how is it being experienced? how is reality being constructed? Subquestions or areas for exploration may be included.

B.   Criteria for research questions

1. Open-ended or "open-beginning"
2. Broad
3. Conducive to context
4. Oriented to people and the human condition

C.   Stating the research question (examples)

1. What is the nature of . . . ?
2. What is the description of . . . ?

   3.   How do people perceive or experience . . . ?
   4.   What is happening here?

IV. HYPOTHESES (QUANTITATIVE)

A. Consists of a conjectural statement of at least one specific relationship between two variables, which can be clearly supported or not supported

B. Criteria for hypotheses

   1.   Delineates a relationship between variables

      — the relationship must be empirically testable through collection of data

   2.   Conditions implicit in the criteria

      — only one relationship may be specified in a single hypothesis
      — the hypothesis must be written before the study is conducted
      — only words describing an empirically testable relationship may be used in a hypothesis

      Ex. Social support will be positively related to patients' psychosocial adjustment to breast cancer.

C. Kinds of hypotheses

   1.   Null hypothesis

      a.   A statement of no relationship
      b.   Denoted as H_0
      c.   If a relationship is found, then H_0 is probably false

   2.   Research hypothesis (directional)

      a.   States the direction that a relationship between two variables is likely to take, meaning that an increase (or decrease) in the independent variable will be related to an increase (or decrease) in the dependent variable
      b.   Used when the investigator is interested only in a relationship manifesting itself in one direction and is willing to "throw away" the results in the other direction, no matter how impressive
      c.   Has some theoretical or empirical rationale for specifying the direction

    d.   Specifies the direction before collecting the data
    e.   Gives direction to the design

> Ex. An increase in deep breathing (X_1) and coughing (X_2) will be related to a decreased need for analgesia (Y_1) and length of hospitalization (Y_2) under the condition of preoperative structured teaching as compared to unstructured teaching.

3.   Research hypothesis (nondirectional)

    a.   States that a relationship exists without indicating directionality
    b.   Often used when there is insufficient empirical evidence in support of a directional hypothesis

> Ex. Patients receiving preoperative instructions differ significantly from patients not receiving preoperative instructions with respect to number of postoperative medication requests.

3

The Literature Review, Definition of Terms, and Theoretical Framework

Literature reviews can be expedited by use of the computer, assistance from a library consultant, and other methods. Often, however, some works cannot be located by any other means than an independent search by the investigator.

In chapter 3, the reader is oriented to the purposes of a literature review and the key sources for locating nursing and nursing-related literature. While technology has facilitated the timely location of studies, and more recently has become a source of secondary reviews and syntheses, investigators need to understand that the evaluation and perspective of someone else is a premise that they are willing to accept. Conversely, the many pieces of information that one obtains from a review of primary studies provides the foundation for identifying or developing a theoretical framework for a quantitative or qualitative study, as well as for making key decisions on other aspects of the study. The reader is urged to set his or her own criteria, given the nature and purpose of the intended study.

Ia. THE LITERATURE REVIEW (QUANTITATIVE)

    A. Primary purposes

        1. Orientation to what is known

            a. Includes identification of assumptions about certain aspects of the phenomenon being studied

        2. Provision of a conceptual or theoretical framework
        3. Indication of a research approach

  a. Research design
  b. Measurement instruments
  c. Statistical analyses

B. Common errors in conducting a literature search that may have implications for the resulting research design

  1. Conducting too cursory a review that overlooks previous studies containing ideas that might improve the proposed research design
  2. Focusing on research findings when reading research reports, thus missing valuable information on methods and measures

Ib. THE LITERATURE REVIEW (QUALITATIVE)

A. Although there are controversial views on conducting a literature review prior to data collection, a preliminary review of the literature for the proposal is useful for a variety of reasons:

  1. Opens the researcher to the complexity of the phenomenon under investigation
  2. Introduces the investigator to the context of the phenomenon and the culture of the participants
  3. Provides additional justification and credibility for the study, e.g., illustrates that this phenomenon has not been studied before or studied in this manner
  4. Signifies how this research will add to extant knowledge

B. It is important that the researcher remain open to the many ideas, hunches, and emerging concepts that may occur during the actual course of the study.
C. In the dissertation, the literature review is far more developed as the findings are compared and contrasted with existing literature and theory.

II. TYPES OF INFORMATION ACQUIRED IN A LITERATURE REVIEW

A. Research findings

  1. Statistical support or refutation

B. Theory (and interpretation)

  1. Broad conceptual issues related to theoretical frameworks for a specific problem
  2. New light on biological or psychological functioning

    C.   Methodologies (research approaches), e.g., *how* the information or findings were found, both quantitative and qualitative

III. SOURCES FOR THE REVIEW

    A. Primary

        1.   Description of an investigation written by the investigator

    B. Secondary

        1.   Description of a study or studies prepared by someone other than the original researcher
        2.   Typically fail to provide sufficient detail about the study
        3.   Rarely possible to achieve complete objectivity in summarizing and reviewing written materials

IV. KEY SOURCES FOR LOCATING NURSING AND NURSING-RELATED LITERATURE

Listed next in alphabetical order is a selection of key sources for researching the nursing and allied health literature fields. Almost all of these sources are currently available in a CD or on-line version, thus making the literature review more efficiently accomplished.

    A. *Cumulative Index to Nursing and Allied Health Literature.* (1977–). Glendale, CA: Glendale Adventist Medical Center Publication Service. ISSN:0888-0530.

        1.   Bimonthly with annual cumulations
        2.   The most important periodical indexing source in the field of nursing
        3.   Contains the *Cumulative Index to Nursing*, 1961–76, Vols. 1–21.
        4.   Covers the major nursing journals as well as selected medical periodicals
        5.   Available on-line

    B. *Dissertation Abstracts International.* (1938–). Ann Arbor, MI: University Microfilms. ISSN:0099-3123.

        1.   Sections A and B are issued monthly, Section C, quarterly
        2.   "[A] compilation of author-prepared abstracts of doctoral dissertations submitted to University Microfilms International for publication in microfilm"

3. Volumes are arranged by topic, with keyword and author indexes
4. Available in various machine readable forms

C. *Health and Psychological Instruments.* (1985–). [computer file]: (HAPI)

   1. CD (developed by the Behavioral Measurements Database Services). Pittsburgh, PA: Behavioral Measurements Database Services.
   2. Semiannual CD product
   3. "[A] database designed to help identify measurement tests used in health, psychological science, organizational behavior, and library and information science; provides source, abstract, and review(s) when applicable"
   4. Each citation gives publication information, an abstract reference, and indicates whether validity and reliability are reported

D. *Hospital and Health Administration Index.* (ca. 1995–). Chicago, IL: American Hospital Association.

   1. Published three times a year, with third issue being a hardbound cumulative volume
   2. Formerly known as *Hospital Literature Index*, 1957–94. ISSN:0018-5736.
   3. "[T]he primary guide to the literature on the organization and administration of hospitals and other health care providers, the financing and delivery of health care, the development and implementation of health policy and reform, and health planning and research"
   4. Emphasizes English-language articles and focuses on industrialized countries, especially the United States
   5. Available on-line via MEDLINE, where it is known as HealthSTAR

E. *Index Medicus.* (1960–). Bethesda, MD: National Library of Medicine. ISSN:0019-3879.

   1. Monthly with annual cumulations
   2. The major English-language indexing source for medical and health-related information
   3. Author, title, and subject indexes cover all aspects of the field
   4. Available on-line as MEDLINE through various vendors
   5. Also includes the *Index to Dental Literature* and the *International Nursing Index*

F. *International Nursing Index.* (1966–). New York: American Journal of Nursing Co. ISSN:0020-8124.

1. Quarterly, the fourth issue being an annual cumulation
2. Published in cooperation with the U.S. National Library of Medicine
3. Covers approximately 200 nursing journals published internationally as well as more than 2,000 titles indexed in *Index Medicus*.
4. Each issue contains a list of serials indexed, new books in nursing, dissertations, and publications of various agencies and organizations
5. Available on-line via MEDLINE

G. *Mental Measurements Year Book* (9th ed.). (1985–). Lincoln, NE: University of Nebraska, Buros Institute of Mental Measurements. Irregular (also available on CD-ROM).

H. *Nursing Research Abstracts*. (1978–). London: Dept. of Health and Social Security Index of Nursing Research. ISSN:0141-3899.

1. Quarterly
2. Focus on British nursing research
3. Contains an author and subject index in each issue
4. Cumulated annually

I. *Nursing Studies Index*. (ca. 1963–72). Philadelphia: Lippincott.

1. Prepared by the Yale University School of Nursing Index Staff, formerly under the direction of Virginia Henderson
2. "[A]n annotated guide to reported studies, research methods, and historical and biographical materials in periodicals, books, and pamphlets published in English"
3. In four volumes: Vol. 1, 1900–29; Vol. 2, 1930–49; Vol. 3, 1950–56; Vol. 4, 1957–59.

J. *Psychological Abstracts*. (1927–). Lancaster, PA: American Psychological Association. ISSN:0033-2887.

1. The index in the field of psychology
2. Indexes more than 1,200 English-language journals and reports
3. Currently also covers books and dissertations
4. Available in various machine readable forms

K. *Science Citation Index*. (1961–). Philadelphia: Institute for Scientific Information. ISSN:0036-8274.

1. An international interdisciplinary index dealing with the literature of science, medicine, agriculture, technology, and the behavioral sciences
2. The concept of citation indexing links current and past publications; thus *Science Citation Index* includes current publications and lists

current works in the *Source Index* by first author. Works cited in the current publications are listed by the first author in the *Citation Index*. A *Permuterm Index* allows subject access to the works in the *Source Index*. A *Corporate Index* lists affiliations of authors listed in the *Source Index*.

    3.   Available on-line as *SciSearch*.

L.   *Social Sciences Citation Index*. (1972–). Philadelphia: Institute for Scientific Information. ISSN:0091-3707.

    1.   Issued three times a year, the third issue being the annual cumulation
    2.   An international interdisciplinary index covering the social, behavioral, and selected fields
    3.   Arrangement and philosophy are the same as *Science Citation Index*, previously cited
    4.   Available on-line as *Social SciSearch*

M.   *Sociological Abstracts* (Vol. 1). (Jan./Oct. 1952/1953). San Diego, CA: Sociological Abstracts, Inc. ISSN:0038-0202.

    1.   Six issues a year
    2.   An international index, each issue of which contains a user's guide, abstracts arranged in classified order and subject, and author and source indexes
    3.   Also included is a section called "International Review of Publications in Sociology" (IRPS), which includes book abstracts and a bibliography of book reviews
    4.   Available in machine readable form

The World Wide Web makes access to information available via the computer. Among the hundreds of sites on the Web that might be useful are:

A.   *The Virginia Henderson Institute and Nursing Library.* http://stti-web. inpui.edu

    1.   The mission is "to provide data, information, knowledge, and communication services to nurses all over the world electronically
    2.   Located at the same site as the *Nursing Research Registry* and contains research that has yet to be published

B.   *The National Library of Medicine.* http://www.nlm.nih.gov

    1.   Contains the NLM on-line catalog, publications, and bibliographies

C. *The National Institutes of Health.* http://www.nih.gov

 1. Health and clinical information, grants and research, molecular biology database, CancerNet, AIDS information, plus access to other NIH sites

D. *Centers for Disease Control.* http://www.cdc.gov

 1. Information on specific diseases, health risks, and prevention, as well as CDC publications

V. METHOD FOR THE REVIEW

A. File cards or computer file according to

 1. sources
 2. subject headings
 3. findings

Note: A *Suggested Guide for Abstracting Research Studies* may be found on p. 60 (Appendix A).

VIa. THEORETICAL FRAMEWORK (QUANTITATIVE)

A. Definitions

 1. Theory

  a. A series of propositions regarding the interrelationships among variables, from which a large number of empirical observations can be deduced
  b. A systematic explanation of some phenomena, broader and more complex than a fact
  c. Identifies the variables needed to explain the phenomena and suggests the nature of the relationships among the variables
  d. Often generates one or more hypotheses to be tested (by deductive logic)

 2. Proposition

  a. A statement indicating a relationship
  b. A set of propositions must form a logically interrelated deductive system, e.g., the theory composed of propositions must provide a mechanism for logically arriving at new statements from the original propositions

3. Axioms

    a. Causal assumptions having the property of a directional relationship. "Select as axioms those propositions that involve variables that are taken to be directly linked causally; axioms should therefore be statements that imply direct causal links among variables" (Blalock, 1969; Dubin, 1969).

4. Variables (see pp. 5–6)
5. Concept

    a. A word that expresses an abstraction formed by generalization from particulars (inductive logic)

6. Construct

    a. A concept
    b. Consciously invented or adapted for a scientific purpose

VIb. THEORETICAL FRAMEWORK (QUALITATIVE)

A. There are contrary views regarding the use of a theoretical framework prior to data collection. Qualitative approaches are used to generate hypotheses and theory rather than to test theory. The theory should emerge from the investigation.

B. If a theoretical perspective is used, it must conform to the philosophical orientations and underpinnings of qualitative research. Examples of appropriate frameworks are:

1. Phenomenology
2. Symbolic interaction
3. Culture
4. History
5. Aesthetics
6. Hermeneutics
7. Chaos theory
8. Ecological psychology
9. Heuristics
10. Ethics

VIIa. DEFINITIONS OF VARIABLES (QUANTITATIVE)

A. There can be no scientific research without observations, and observations are not possible without clear and specific instructions on what and how to observe.

1. Serve as bridges between the theory-hypothesis level and the level of observation
2. Enable the researcher to measure variables

B. Both conceptual and operational definitions are important.

  1. Conceptual definition

     a. A definition that defines a construct with other constructs
     b. A variable may be defined by using other words
     c. A variable may be defined by specifying what actions or behaviors the variable expresses or implies

  2. Operational definition

     a. A definition that assigns meaning to a construct or a variable by specifying the activities or operations necessary to measure the construct or variable

VIIb. DEFINITIONS (QUALITATIVE)

In qualitative research, there are no a priori definitions of the phenomenon under study. Definitions emerge from the inquiry as themes, descriptions of the phenomenon, depictions of meaning, and portrayals of experiences. In grounded theory, definitions of the theoretical concepts and their relationships are an outcome of the study.

Note: A *Guide to Critique of Quantitative Research*, two exemplar articles with critiques, and an article for practice may be found in Appendix B (pp. 62–101). In Appendix C (pp. 102–119), the *Guide to Critique of Qualitative Research* may be found, along with an exemplar article with a critique and a practice article. It is suggested that the reader use the guides and exemplar articles as illustrations of the content of the present document.

4

Research Designs

The issue of which design is appropriate to answer a particular research question is relatively complex. Within the "rough" categories of "quantitative" and "qualitative" designs are many designs with specific characteristics. A basic understanding of these characteristics is important in selecting a design that (1) has the potential for answering the research question, (2) is relatively precise and efficient, and (3) will produce valid and reliable results.

The major characteristics of qualitative designs are reviewed in this chapter. Characteristics of quantitative designs also are discussed, along with suggestions for selection. Since many books and courses are available on research designs, chapter 4 is intended only as a point of departure in seeking more in-depth information.

Most research is expensive in terms of time, effort, and possibly funds. Thus it is essential that the design be selected and implemented with care. The standards for quantitative and qualitative designs are rigorous. If these issues are not taken seriously, the investigator may (1) encounter costly problems during the study, (2) be unable to complete the research, or (3) not know how to interpret the findings.

I.   THE RESEARCH DESIGN

The research design provides a plan that governs the conduct of the research and is a function of the research question(s) to be answered. Research questions may generate from nursing practice, an extant theory, a theoretical framework developed from the scientific literature, conceptual models, or the literature.

A.   Types of research designs (quantitative)

1.   Descriptive
2.   Experimental
3.   Quasi-experimental
4.   Correlational

B.   Types of research designs (qualitative)

    1.   Phenomenology
    2.   Grounded theory
    3.   Ethnography
    4.   Case study
    5.   Historiography
    6.   Hermeneutics
    7.   Ethnomethodology
    8.   Critical or emancipatory research
    9.   Action research
   10.   Foundational inquiry or philosophical analysis

IIa.   THE RESEARCH DESIGN (QUANTITATIVE)

A.   Characteristics and aims of the quantitative design

    1.   Descriptive

       a.   Obtain information on topics for which there is little previous investigation
       b.   Describe events as they exist naturally
       c.   No introduction of anything new
       d.   No modification or control of the situation being studied

    2.   Experimental

       a.   Determine whether or not a predicted result occurs when a specified action is taken
       b.   Conducted under a controlled situation

          — some factors are held constant
          — other factors are manipulated
          — random sampling and assignment to groups
          — the results in the manipulated situation are evaluated and compared with those observed in the controlled situation

    3.   Quasi-experimental

       a.   Attempt to approximate a true experimental design when certain characteristics of a true experimental design cannot be attained, e.g., the researcher is not able to

          — randomly sample

      — manipulate factors
      — control when or to whom the experimental treatment will be introduced

4. Correlational

    a. Exploration of relationships among variables
    b. Regression studies are a special case of correlational designs

      — the researcher attempts to explain or predict changes in one variable (criterion) on the basis of changes in the other factors (predictors)

B. Sampling in quantitative designs (see chapter 5)
C. Measurement in quantitative designs (see chapters 7 and 8)
D. Protection of human subjects

    1. Discuss the nature of participation in the study and reinforce by a written description
    2. Assure that consent or refusal will not affect health care (if appropriate)
    3. Explain procedures for assurance of confidentiality or anonymity
    4. State that withdrawal from the study at any time is permitted without repercussions
    5. Develop a mechanism by which results of the study will be provided

IIb. THE RESEARCH DESIGN (QUALITATIVE)

A. Characteristics of research designs and approaches (qualitative)

There are a variety of designs and approaches in qualitative research. The following are descriptions of some of the more common ones and "central questions" (Patton, 1990, p. 88) that the approach raises.

1. Phenomenology

    a. Involves understanding the essence of a phenomenon
    b. Describes the "lived experience from the perception of those experiencing it"
    c. Asks, "What is the structure and essence of experience of this phenomenon for these people?" (p. 88)
    d. Emanates from phenomenological philosophy
    e. For example, *The experience of alienation in nursing home residents: A phenomenological inquiry*

2. Grounded theory

    a. Develop or generate a theory grounded in or derived from empirical data to explain a phenomenon or social or psychological process

    b. Emanates from sociology or symbolic interactionism

    c. For example, *Negotiating in interdisciplinary teams: A grounded theory*

3. Ethnography

    a. Study of cultures and "life ways" of people

    b. Asks, "What is the culture of this group of people?" (p. 88)

    c. Emanates from social and behavioral sciences

    d. For example, *Bodymindspirit: Understanding the culture of holistic practitioners*

4. Case study

    a. A holistic, detailed, and in-depth exploration of an individual, a group as an entity, an organization, or an event in context, conducted in natural, real-life situations. Emanates from social and behavioral sciences

    b. For example, *The family experience with multiple births: A case study*

5. Historiography

    a. Investigates, analyzes, interprets, and narrates past events through a critical examination and synthesis of historical evidence, such as documents, artifacts, personal accounts

    b. Emanates from history

    c. For example, *A history of the NYU Division of Nursing from 1960–1975*

6. Hermeneutics

    a. The art of interpretation in context so that text, human acts, or outcomes can be understood

    b. Asks, "What are the conditions under which a human act took place or a product was produced that make it possible to interpret its meaning?" (p. 88)

    c. Emanates from philosophy, theology, and literary criticism

    d. For example, *The language of caring in the nursing literature:*

An hermeneutical analysis

7. Ethnomethodology

 a. Focus on people's understandings, the routine of the common social world
 b. Asks, "How do people make sense of their everyday activities so as to behave in socially acceptable ways?" (p. 88)
 c. For example, *A study of the meaning of life in a wheelchair*

8. Critical or emancipatory research

 a. Attempts to surface and expose injustice and oppression within the context of the empowerment and emancipation of people
 b. Emanates from critical theory and postmodern social theory
 c. For example, *Hidden lives: Giving voice to sexually abused adolescents*

9. Action research

 a. Practice oriented research that is conducted in collaboration with participants in a program, organization or community
 b. Incorporates data collection and problem identification, planning, implementing and evaluating changes to solve problems and improve a specific system
 c. Emanates from social and action theory
 d. For example, *Funded research on women's health problems: Inquiry for change*

10. Foundational inquiry or philosophical analysis

 a. "Used to articulate, clarify, and refine basic conceptualizations" (Edgerton, 1988, p. 176).

 — done through philosophical analysis, a method of reflection and argumentation, leading to the "clarification of the language of a science" demonstrating the "possible reconciliation of apparently different concepts" (Manchester, 1988, p. 241), and reconceptualizations to increase the consistency between conceptual foundations or assumptions and particular scientific frameworks.

 b. For example, *A philosophical analysis of suffering*

B.   Characteristics of the qualitative design

1.   The design is flexible. It emerges as understanding increases; the specifics of the approach evolve as the inquiry proceeds.
2.   The research process proceeds in a spiral, looping, cyclic fashion. Data collection and data analysis are blended, occur simultaneously, and inform one another.
3.   The sample is usually small and emphasizes depth versus breadth.
4.   The sample is chosen purposively or theoretically versus randomly or by convenience, and is selected serially, e.g., who and what come subsequently depend on who and what came before.
5.   There is a partner relationship between the researcher and the participant or "knower" of the phenomenon.
6.   Two primary techniques are used in gathering data: participant observation and in-depth, unstructured interviewing. Other techniques include the use of videotapes, photographs, projective techniques, life histories, kinesics, and analysis of various documents.
7.   Data are gathered over time. There is prolonged engagement in the field.
8.   Data analysis focuses on discovery of patterns, description, and interpretation of the data to "make meaning."
9.   Analysis and conclusions are directly supported by (grounded in) the actual data.
10. Qualitative analysis is usually presented in narrative rather than numerical form.
11. Qualitative inquiry necessitates a continuous and honest exploration of the researcher's own values and ethical orientations. The researcher brackets preconceived notions, beliefs, attitudes, values, and knowledge about the phenomenon to "see" and "hear" the experience of the other.

C.   Qualitative design or approach—general

1.   Used to orient the reader

a.   Purpose of the approach
b.   Philosophical assumptions of the approach
c.   Background or foundation of the approach
d.   Definitions of the terms of the approach
e.   Process and procedures of the approach
f.   Result of the approach—what will it produce, and why is this important in this study?

D.   Qualitative design or approach—specific

1. This activity is the application of the specific design or approach as implemented in this study. It is a thorough explication of the details of this study.

    a. Repeat the purpose of the study and the research question
    b. Describe how each process will be carried out in this study (with the understanding that the design is flexible and may change as the inquiry progresses)
    c. Include a time line

E. Sample—participants

1. This is a description of the sample or unit of analysis (individual, group, culture, event, or process).

    a. Describe the setting; give rationale for the setting
    b. Identify the sampling method (purposive/selective or theoretical) and describe sampling procedure
    c. Describe how entrée to the setting, both official and informal, will be gained
    d. Describe how saturation will be achieved (continuation of sampling to the point of redundancy until no new or disconfirming information or evidence is found)

F. Data Collection

Data for qualitative inquiries come from various sources: observations, interviews, verbal reports, documents, pictures, diaries, and artifacts.

1. Participant observation

    a. "A period of intense social interaction between the researcher and [participants], in the milieu of the latter. During this period, data are unobtrusively and systematically collected" (Bogdan & Taylor, 1975, p. 5). The researcher is an involved observer, taking part in some activities while carefully observing the situation to record and analyze what is occurring.
    b. The researcher observes people, setting, atmosphere, activities, interactions and dialogue, events, context, and responses to the researcher.
    c. The researcher must consider the role of the observer, characterization of the researcher's role to others, depiction of the research purpose to others, duration of the observations, and focus of the observations (Patton, 1990).

      d.   The researcher looks for who is present, what is happening, when activities occur, where they occur, why things happen, and how things happen.

      e.   Informal interviewing often is used for participant clarification, explanation, or expansion.

  2.   In-depth or unstructured interviewing

      a.   "A conversation with a purpose," which should produce interesting and prolific stories, data that are abundant in detail and examples, and narratives that reveal people's complex feelings, perceptions, and viewpoints.

      b.   The researcher should have an interview guide of five to six questions with which to begin the interview.

      c.   Questions may change as data are analyzed and other areas take on importance.

      d.   Follow-up questions are used to increase more detailed inquiry.

  3.   Discuss the details and procedures of data gathering techniques, e.g., how conducted, when, where, with whom, approximate time per data collection sessions, use of tape recorder and transcriber.

  4.   Describe the data records to be used for the study

      a.   Field notes—detailed recordings of a variety of information collected in the field. These can be descriptive and reflective

      b.   Interview transcripts

      c.   Personal and methodological journal—the personal/methodological notes taken during the inquiry, including the researcher's ideas about the project, uniqueness of the method, methodological issues and how they were handled, and the researcher's feelings about the study, participants, assumptions, reactions, and the researcher's frame of mind at the time

      d.   Analytic log—the researcher's theoretical notes, analytic memos, and conceptualizations over the course of the inquiry, including interpretations, conjectures, inferences and speculations about what is being learned and the emerging patterns, themes, and concepts

  5.   Discuss how and where the data will be stored

  6.   Discuss anticipated problems in data collection and the potential researcher's effect on the design

G.   Protection of human subjects

1. Discuss informed consent and how anonymity and confidentiality of the participants are to be ensured
2. Address human subjects' review, both at the university if indicated and the settings in which the study will take place
3. Consider potential ethical dilemmas when observing or interviewing about sensitive topics
4. Identify referral sources if the nature of the inquiry potentially may be upsetting to the participant
5. Consider how negotiations will be handled

III. FACTORS AFFECTING THE SELECTION OF A RESEARCH DESIGN

A. The research question(s)

1. Generally, there are several designs that can be employed in studying a given broad research problem.
2. Alternative designs that are equally valid for investigating a problem are rarely equally efficient.

B. Knowledge of the research topic
C. Knowledge of different kinds of designs
D. Application of criteria for selecting a design

1. Has the potential for answering the research question (and testing the hypotheses in the case of a quantitative design)
2. Relatively precise and efficient
3. Affords utilization of powerful statistical procedures if the design is quantitative
4. Economical for the researcher and the subjects
5. Produces valid and reliable results
6. Allows an opportunity for comparison of study findings with the results of other investigations
7. Conforms to accepted procedures used in research on the designated topic

IVa. QUANTITATIVE DESIGNS—INTERNAL AND EXTERNAL VALIDITY

In research, the researcher attempts to determine if the variable studied is actually the "causal" factor or if there are extraneous or intervening variables unaccounted for in the study setting. In other words, in studying the relationship between an independent and a dependent variable, one is hypothesizing that the independent variable is related to the occurrence of the dependent variable. But is X always the factor that operates in the occurrence of Y? Or is there an extraneous, or intervening, variable confounding the situation?

Internal validity addresses the question of whether the researchers are measuring what they think they are. External validity is the extent to which the researcher can then make a generalization about the relationships identified in the experimental setting. Internal validity is achieved primarily by means of a good research design with maximum controls. External validity is more difficult to achieve than internal validity because subjects usually cannot be selected at random from a defined population.

Ex.   Is preoperative structured teaching truly related to postoperative recovery, or are there factors other than teaching playing a role in the results?

Note: A discussion of the design and methods for control of extraneous variables for this study may be found in Appendix E (pp. 121–123).

A.   Threats to validity

Source	Definition
history	the effect of events that occur simultaneously with the investigation
maturation	changes in the subject as the result of conditions, such as fatigue
regression toward the mean	a group chosen because of its extreme position on a continuum will tend to exhibit movement toward the mean on retest
testing	the effect of one test on a subsequent test as the result of practice, memory, or training
instrumentation	the effect of variations in accuracy or efficiency of an instrument from time to time or from one condition to another
differential selection of subjects	selection of two or more groups that are not comparable on some crucial variable that may bias the outcome
subject mortality	the effect of differential losses from groups so that the final result is to render them not comparable

B.   Strategies for control

1.   In developing the theoretical rationale, consider the dependent variable and try to identify other variables that are related to it.

2. Control the variables that are not under study but that may contribute substantially to the variance in the dependent variable(s).
3. Maximize the experimental variable, e.g., make sure it will operate.
4. Consider selecting a sample that controls for the extraneous variables, e.g., a sample that is homogeneous for those variables.
5. Use random selection or random assignment for experimental and quasi-experimental designs whenever possible.

   a. True randomization permits one to say that experimental groups are equal at the outset, e.g., it theoretically controls for extraneous variables
   b. Although randomization cannot always be achieved, care needs to be taken in assessing the similarity of groups

6. An extraneous variable may be built into the design, e.g., measured, permitting the calculation of variance in the dependent variable that may be attributed to the variable.
7. Subjects in the control and experimental groups may be matched for specific variables.
8. Control the testing situation.
9. Minimize errors of testing.

5

Sampling in Quantitative Designs:
Basic Issues and Concepts

The sampling procedure is a very important part of the research design. The careful observation of principles for drawing a sample, depending on the design to be used, is directly related to the internal and external validity of the study. In this chapter, Dr. Joseph Giacquinta, professor at New York University and expert on sampling methods, provides content on sampling error and bias that can occur if specific principles are not followed. Sampling frames and styles of sampling are discussed with excellent examples. Guides for determining sample size are offered, as well as general sampling suggestions.

I. INTERNAL AND EXTERNAL VALIDITY OF QUANTITATIVE STUDIES

As noted, internal validity means whether or not the results of a specific empirical study are accurate for the sample used in the investigation. External validity means whether or not valid sample results can be generalized to the larger population from which the sample was taken. They depend on the problem formation, measurement, statistical analysis, and sampling design.

A. Sampling principles and concepts

1. Developed most fully within the tradition of survey research
2. Experimental designs depend more on relatively small, convenience, or sometimes purposive samples due to

a. unavailability of large numbers of representative, willing subjects
b. practicality of administering treatments to large numbers of subjects
c. need for random assignment of subjects from the available sample

pool to either an experimental or control group, thereby equating the two groups

B. Quasi-experimental designs pose even greater strains on the principles of proper sampling

    1. Internal and external validity are more difficult to assess
    2. Experimenter frequently has no control over

        a. the source of subjects
        b. the size of the sample
        c. whether the subjects are in the experimental or control group
        d. the nature and administration of the treatment

II. SAMPLING ERROR AND SAMPLING BIAS

A. Sampling error

    1. Deviations from true population parameters, e.g., population means, standard deviations, percentages, correlations, that result from the study of just one sample taken from that population
    2. Probable error despite the fact that the sample was scientifically drawn
    3. Can be estimated
    4. A direct function of the size of a *properly* drawn sample
    5. Within limits, the larger the sample drawn, the smaller the probable error

Note: Formulas for calculating standard sampling error may be obtained from Salant and Dillman (1994) or Henry (1990).

B. Sample bias

    1. Difficult to estimate in advance largely due to

        a. the way in which a sample is selected
        b. whether the subjects fully cooperate

    2. Methods for avoidance

        a. Draw a *representative* sample
        b. Strive for as much cooperation as possible

            Ex. Low sample returns (if a mail questionnaire is used) or low sample cooperation (if phone or in-person interviews are conducted) signal that the sample statistics deviate in critical ways from the true population values.

III. FIVE LEVELS OF SAMPLING REALITY AND THEIR POTENTIAL IMPACT ON INTERNAL AND EXTERNAL VALIDITY

A. Identifying the ideal population of interest

   1. Directly connected to a research problem, e.g., practicing nurses or hospital patients

B. Delimiting a subpopulation

   1. The sample seldom remains at a general level, e.g., delimitations are consciously stated or implicit

      Ex. Patients that are males suffering from cancer and are in a hospice care setting

   2. Insufficient delimitation leads to both unacceptable sampling error and bias

C. Locating a sampling frame

   1. Should be a fair reflection of the delimited population
   2. Sample from that frame by using some proper procedure such as simple random sampling or systematic sampling
   3. Available sampling frame may not reflect the desired population as delimited, leading to sample bias

D. Drawing the sample

   1. Some, if not many, of the subjects in the selected sample may fail to cooperate
   2. Sample size may be inadequate, leading to

      a. larger than acceptable sampling error

E. Studying the sample

   1. Sample size may be less representative than the one originally drawn, leading to

      a. potential sample bias

2. Sample returned may be too small a proportion of that drawn and contacted, leading to

    a. unacceptable sampling error

    b. sample bias

IV. SAMPLING: SOURCES OF FRAMES, STYLES OF SAMPLING, AND SAMPLE SIZE

  A. Sources and availability of sampling frames

    1. Depends on the delimited population as specified by the research design

      Exs. —membership lists of social groupings
          —work rosters of organizations that contain the names of persons who fit the delimited population

    2. Information about the sampling units are preferable to those that contain simply names and addresses

      a. Permits comparison of subjects who cooperated with those who chose not to cooperate

      b. Sheds light on the possibility of sampling bias introduced by noncooperation and the extent to which the sample drawn is representative of the larger frame

  B. Styles of sampling

    1. Simple random sampling

      a. Basic approach upon which statistical significance testing and the assessment of confidence intervals are based

      b. Tests of statistical significance, e.g., the t test, the F test, or chi square, indicate how frequently the results obtained from a study occur by chance

      c. Based on sample statistics, a confidence interval indicates the range of scores within which the true population value most probably falls

      d. Proper technique ensures that all subjects in a sampling frame have an equal chance of being selected

      e. Every unit is assigned a number

      f. From a table of random numbers, subject IDs are selected until the desired number of units is reached

2. Systematic sampling

    a. Every nth subject is taken from an unnumbered sampling frame until the desired quantity of subjects is selected

    b. Unacceptable if there are repeated patterns in the listing, e.g., names listed on each page are rank ordered in some way

    c. Economical in terms of time

3. Stratified sampling

    a. Ensures *inclusion* of certain characteristics of a sample and/or *exclusion* of others

    b. Useful when the researcher wants to include certain characteristics in the sample in proportion to their presence in the larger population or disproportionately so

        Ex. If only males are to be studied, a sampling frame also containing females would have to be stratified according to gender and then limited to the selection of males only. If the males and females were to be compared, even though the researcher is sampling from a frame of elderly bedridden patients (usually composed of more females than males), then a disproportionately larger number of males and disproportionately smaller number of females would have to be selected to have an equal number of both sexes. If one were interested in certain matters related to the overall population of elderly, bedridden patients, then after stratifying according to gender, males and females would have to be selected in numbers proportionate to their presence in the larger elderly population. The selection within each stratum could be accomplished by simple random sampling or systematically if the available list were in an unbiased form, e.g., alphabetical.

4. Cluster sampling

    a. Used when there is an absence of an adequate frame for subjects

        Ex. In studying hospital nurses, one might have a list of hospitals in a certain area, but not the nurses within them. One way, therefore, to select nurses would be to select a few hospitals and then study all the nurses within them. Another would be to select hospitals, then floors within them, then study all the nurses on the selected floors.

5. Quota sampling

    a. Useful when the research involves face-to-face interviews requiring the specification of a number of persons possessing particular characteristics, e.g., 20 females under 30 years of age who jog, 10 males over 40 who smoke, and

    b. When there is no clear sampling frame but a physical place where subjects can be located

        Ex. Interview of patients attending a particular clinic

6. Snowball sampling

    a. Useful in situations where no actual sampling frame exists, and

    b. When few desired subjects are known

    c. The investigator starts with the few known subjects and from them attempts to connect with still others of the same kind until the desired sample size is reached

7. Convenience sampling

    a. Uses whatever cooperative subjects are easily at hand

    b. Because of the way the subjects were selected, their representativeness is in question

C. Sample size and methods to determine the minimum needed

1. General rules

    a. For survey and correlational research, draw as large a sample as is financially possible, within certain limits

    b. Generally, sample sizes larger than 1,000 to 1,200 subjects from populations of more than 100,000 are unnecessary since the increased accuracy of the statistics gained from larger samples does not justify the larger numbers and costs

    c. Samples smaller than 200 or 300 subjects usually lead to confidence intervals that are too wide to be satisfying and also limit the kinds of subsample analyses that may be necessary

2. Methods to determine sample size

    a. Power analysis if

        — the effect size can be specified

        — some judgment about sample variances can be made

Note: See Cohen (1988) or Light, Singer, and Willett (1990) for information.

b. Standard error formulas if

— the researcher wants to be 95% sure that the true percentage or correlation falls within a limited range of plus or minus a few percentage points or correlational points

c. Rules of thumb—informal standards that over time have come to be accepted by professionals in various fields but typically are not easily traced to their original sources

Exs: —20 to 30 subjects for each independent variable if the fundamental statistical analysis is to be multiple regression —a minimum of 5 subjects for each item if factor analyses are to be done

d. Other factors

— the greater the homogeneity of the population, the smaller the size of the sample needed
— if the study is theory building, a smaller sample is required than if the purpose is theory testing or descriptive of a large population
— the more variables and delimitations, the greater the need for larger numbers since comparisons of subgroups and combinations of variables necessitate larger numbers
— if a sampling frame contains a large number of subjects who are no longer available, then a much larger number will be needed to reach the minimal size originally calculated

V. GENERAL SAMPLING SUGGESTIONS

A. Know as much as possible about the population and sampling frame.
B. Find and use a sampling frame that is representative or clearly heuristic, given the research interest, that has more than names and addresses associated with it
C. Use sound sampling procedures, e.g., stratified random sampling.
D. Within limits, draw as large a sample as is technically and financially feasible.
E. Use follow-up procedures to achieve as high a return rate of questionnaires as possible or to gain the cooperation of phone or in-person interviewees.

6

Data Analysis and Interpretation

The analyses and interpretation of data collected in quantitative and qualitative designs have significant differences. Both contribute a great deal to the knowledge base of nursing science, which has as a primary purpose excellence in patient care. Clearly, health care is increasingly influenced by the demand for universal access to care, cost containment, and public policy. As part of health care reform and managed care, outcomes of care that can be documented are receiving increased attention. Thus the findings and outcomes from nursing studies need to be evaluated for their potential to improve practice as well as for such criteria as internal and external validity.

The purposes and processes of quantitative and qualitative data analyses are outlined in this chapter. Similar to the description of internal and external validity for quantitative designs in chapter 5, the criteria for quality, or rigor, in qualitative research are described. Whether the reader's purpose is to design a study or evaluate a study for application to practice, a basic knowledge of analyses and interpretation is essential for making such informed decisions.

Ia. DATA ANALYSIS AND INTERPRETATION (QUANTITATIVE)

    A.   Statistical methods should be appropriate to the level of data collected. Interval and ordinal data are most often encountered in the behavioral sciences.

    B.   Kinds of data

          1.   Nominal

               a.   Lowest level of measurement or means of classifying data
               b.   Consists of classifying observations into categories

                    — categories are mutually exclusive, e.g., each observation must be capable of classification into one and only one category

    — any nominal variable may be dichotomized and then treated as a binary variable, assigning a *1* to members of one group and a *0* to the other

2.   Ordinal

   a.   Distinguished from nominal data by the property of order among the categories
   b.   Categories may be thought of as higher than or lower than the adjacent category
   c.   No specification of the magnitude of the interval between two categories

3.   Interval

   a.   Distinguished from ordinal data by having equal intervals between the units of measure, e.g., a score of 50 points is halfway between 40 and 60
   b.   A true quantitative score
   c.   Lacks a true zero, e.g., one cannot interpret a score of 50 as indicating twice as much of a given trait or ability as 25

4.   Ratio

   a.   Possesses all properties of interval scales
   b.   Has a true zero

C.   Nonparametric statistical procedures are indicated for nominal and ordinal data, e.g., chi square. Parametric statistics are intended for interval and ratio data, e.g., Pearson product moment correlation coefficient.

D.   Descriptive statistics (used to describe data)

Descriptive statistics indicate the central tendency of scores, e.g., where the scores tend to group together, and the variability of scores, e.g., how far the scores spread from the center of the distribution of scores.

1.   Measures of central tendency

   a.   Mean

       — one of the most commonly used measures of central tendency
       — the arithmetic average of a set of data

$$\text{Mean} = \frac{sum\ of\ x}{n}$$

b.   Median

    —   the midpoint in a set of ranked scores (highest to lowest), e.g., the same number of scores are above the midpoint as below

    —   if there is an even number of scores, the midpoint score is interpolated, e.g., a midpoint of 10 is interpolated for the set 5, 6, 7, 9, 11, 12, 12, 14 even though the score of 10 was not attained

c.   Mode

    —   consists of the most frequently occurring score in a distribution of scores

    —   usually located near the center of the distribution

    —   a less frequently used index of central tendency

2.   Guide to selection of measure of central tendency

    a.   Mean

       —   the only measure that uses all the data, e.g., all scores are used in computing the mean

       —   provides the more sensitive index of central tendency

       —   more stable statistically

       —   when there are one or two extreme scores, however, the mean does not provide an accurate reflection of the average

    b.   Median

       —   not influenced by extreme scores

       —   a good index of central tendency when working with sets of data that depart from normal distributions, e.g., there is an extremely high proportion of superior scores and a low proportion of extremely inferior scores

    c.   Mode

       —   an easily located measure of central tendency

3.   Measures of variability

In addition to measures of central tendency, it is desirable to have a measure of how the data are dispersed in either direction from the center of a distribution of scores

a. Range

— most easily calculated measure of variability
— obtained by subtracting the lowest score value from the highest

b. Variance

— reflects distance of the individual scores from the mean
— calculation

$$\text{variance} = \frac{sum\ of\ x^2}{n},$$

where sum of x^2 = sum of squared deviations from the mean, and n = the number of cases in the distribution

c. Standard deviation

— consists of the square root of the variance
— is used to describe variability when the mean is used to describe central tendency
— while the mean is an average of the scores of a set, the standard deviation is a sort of average of how distant the individual scores in a distribution are removed from the mean itself

E. Inferential statistics

a. More complex than descriptive methods and, in most instances, make use of descriptive statistics, e.g., mean and standard deviation
b. Describe data in hand, e.g., from the sample

— test for differences, as in differences between means of two groups (*t* test)
— test for relationships between variables (correlation)
— make predictions regarding a subject's performance on one variable, given the performance on another (regression)
— test for significant differences between means of two or more groups (analysis of variance)

      c.   Allow one to draw inferences from sample data that have wider generalizability

F.   It is crucial to accept as tenable those hypotheses that are true and to reject those that are false

    1.   The null hypothesis

        a.   A commonly used method of stating hypotheses in research

            —   postulates that there is no (null) relationship between the variables under study

        b.   The research hypothesis

            —   a positive statement of the null hypothesis

    2.   Acceptance or rejection of hypotheses is based on

        a.   statistical significance
        b.   power
        c.   effect size, and
        d.   sample size

Note: An explanation of the testing of an hypothesis, with an exemplar study, may be found in Appendix F (pp. 000–000). The explanation includes the concepts of statistical significance, error, directionality, and power.

Fill ɪɪо.

Ib. DATA ANALYSIS AND INTERPRETATION (QUALITATIVE)

A.   Analysis is the investigator's attempt to discover and abstract meaning. It is creative and interactive, requiring much time, critical thinking, and emotional and conceptual energy.

B.   Purposes

    1.   To explore and describe

        a.   Gain understanding about a particular phenomenon or group of individuals

    2.   To discover and explain

        a.   Search the data to discover underlying themes, core patterns, and concepts that become the basis for inferences, interpretations,

and generating hypothetical statements about the meaning of the phenomenon
b. Analysis can be furthered to construct an explanatory scheme, model, or substantive grounded theory

3. Extend an existing theory to a grand or formal theory or to other contexts or other conditions

C. Analytic approaches

1. There are numerous approaches to analyzing qualitative data. Tesch (1990) identifies approximately 26 approaches to qualitative research, each having a somewhat different approach to analysis (Mariano, 1995).

   Exs. analytic induction, content/textual analysis, thematic analysis, matrix analysis, constant comparison, phenomenological analysis, quasi-judicial analysis, and discourse analysis

2. There are guidelines for data analysis, however, because each qualitative inquiry is distinctive: The analytical methods used will be unique depending on the skills, insights, analytic abilities, and style of the investigator.

D. Elements of qualitative analysis

1. Data analysis and data collection occur concurrently informing one another
2. The investigator becomes immersed in and dwells within the data
3. The researcher divides the data into smaller units for analysis, e.g., coding and categorizing, and then reintegrates them into a conceptual whole, the result being a higher order synthesis
4. Interpretation is required, making inferences, assigning meanings, speculating, abstracting understandings, offering explications, and dealing with disconfirming evidence, differences in data, and rival hypotheses—all to test the feasibility of an interpretation
5. There is a balance between the interpretations made and the data or evidence that serves as the support for the interpretations. Conclusions are directly grounded in description, quotations, or documentary evidence

E. Processes of qualitative analysis

1. Reflection in analysis is personal and data oriented

a. Personal reflection

— feelings, assumptions, preconceived ideas, reactions, values explored and bracketed as necessary so that analysis is not merely a projection of what the researcher believes, thinks, or feels

b. Data-oriented reflection

— the researcher interrogates, contemplates, dialogues with, and critically appraises the data

2. Comparison is used in disclosing conceptual similarities and differences, generating themes and patterns, contrasting themes and patterns across individual cases and sites
3. Creativity is used in making sense of the data

a. Use of metaphor, analogy, imagery

4. Theoretical sensitivity provides meaning and understanding

a. Achieved by

— continual verification of hunches and hypotheses with the active data
— maintenance of a skeptical stance
— familiarity with the literature
— adherence to sound research practices

F. Description of the process of data analysis

1. State exactly what will be done in the study

a. Depending on the method of analysis, will there be coding, categorizing, use of matrices, constant comparison, writing memos, sorting, and making use of the literature?

2. State how the framework will inform the analysis of the study
3. Describe the use of the computer software packages for data management

Ic. CRITERIA FOR QUALITY AND RIGOR IN QUALITATIVE RESEARCH

Measures need to be identified to ensure trustworthiness of the inquiry.

A. Credibility—assurance of plausible interpretations and conclusions

    1. Prolonged engagement in the field or setting
    2. Triangulation of data sources, e.g., use of a variety of sources
    3. Ongoing peer review
    4. Negative case analysis, e.g., search and account for disconfirming data
    5. Member checking, e.g., having the participants review and confirm the researcher's interpretations and conclusions

B. Transferability—permits someone else to decide if the findings of the inquiry are applicable in another setting

    1. Provision of a detailed database and "thick" description

C. Dependability—determination of the reliability of the findings that enables someone else to logically follow the process and procedures of the inquiry

    1. Use of an auditor to inspect the inquiry process as well as the records relating to the inquiry to judge its authenticity

D. Confirmability—affirmation that the findings, conclusions, and recommendations are supported by or grounded in the data and there is concordance between the researcher's interpretations and the actual evidence

    1. Use of an audit procedure
    2. Use of a reflexive journal

E. Evaluative qualities of qualitative inquiry (Mariano, 1995).

    1. Verity—Does the work ring true, and is it intellectually honest?
    2. Integrity—Is the work structurally sound, and is the research rationale logical and appropriate?
    3. Rigor—Is there depth of intellect rather than simplistic, superficial reasoning?
    4. Utility—Is the work useful and professionally relevant, and does it make a contribution?
    5. Vitality—Is the work meaningful, providing a sense of vibrancy and discovery, and do the metaphors communicate forcefully?
    6. Aesthetics—Is the work enriching, and does it touch the spirit and give others insight into some universal part of themselves?

7

Principles of Measurement

Measurement is an issue in any research. The spectrum of measurement extends from the nondirected interview used in qualitative research to the highly structured, self-administered Likert scales that are scored. A full description of the many kinds of measurements, or observations, is beyond the scope of this book. Thus an outline of the principles of quantitative measurement is provided and the various kinds of measurement tools are described. These include the commonly used interviews and questionnaires, scales and other psychological measures, observational methods, and vignettes. Suggestions are provided for locating an appropriate measure for a study and assessing its validity and reliability. For a more comprehensive discussion of measurement issues, the reader is referred to the many texts on psychometric theory and measurement.

I. METHODS OF MEASUREMENT

    A. Measurement consists of objective methods of observation

        1. Those in which anyone following prescribed rules will assign the same ratings, or "scores," to what is observed
        2. Agreement among observers is at a maximum
        3. All methods of observation are inferential, e.g., inferences about attitudes or behaviors of individuals are made on the basis of the ratings assigned to items on specific forms of measurement instruments

            a. Interviews, questionnaires
            b. Scales, tests, and other psychological measures
            c. Observational methods
            d. Vignettes

    B. Interviews and questionnaires

1. The interview

   a. A direct method of obtaining information
   b. May be used to study relationships and to test hypotheses
   c. When used in research to test hypotheses

      — The questions, their sequence and wording are fixed
      — The interview must be carefully constructed and pretested
      — The interview schedule must be subjected to the same criteria of reliability, validity, and objectivity as any other measuring instrument

2. The questionnaire

   a. Differs from interviews in that they are self-administered and highly structured

C. Scales and other psychological measures

   1. The test

      a. A systematic procedure in which the subject is presented with a set of items to which he or she responds
      b. The examiner assigns a rating, or score, to each response
      c. Inferences are made about the subject's possession of whatever the test is designed to measure
      d. A trait, attitude, or emotion can be measured and quantified in this manner

   2. The scale

      a. A set of response symbols for each item that permits the assignment of a rating according to rules

Ex.	Strongly agree	5
	Agree	4
	Undecided	3
	Disagree	2
	Strongly disagree	1

      b. Assignment and totaling of the values or ratings indicate the degree to which the subject possesses the characteristic that the scale measures
      c. Takes advantage of any intensity structure that may exist among the individual items

Ex. A measure of attitude toward research

Research is essential to the generation of new knowledge.
SA   A   U   D   SD

Nursing research is a key factor in developing and evaluating practice.
SA   A   U   D   SD

Participation in conducting research is a responsibility of all members of the profession.
SA   A   U   D   SD

Professional nurses should allocate time to research activities even if it requires use of their free time.
SA   A   U   D   SD

Presumably, if respondents agree with the content in one item, they are in agreement with all items preceding it in the list, e.g., those with lesser intensities.

D. Observational methods

1. A direct observation of behavior

   a. The investigator assigns values to behavioral acts, or sequences of acts, according to rules to obtain reliable and objective observations from which inferences may be drawn
   b. Requires an operational definition of what one is observing
   c. Behaviors must be assigned to categories that are mutually exclusive
   d. Units of behavior must be determined (molar versus molecular)
   e. Sampling, or when and how the observations will be made, must be decided (event sampling, time sampling)
   f. The nature of the relationship between the observer and subjects needs to be defined. Concealment refers to the degree to which subjects are aware that they are being observed; intervention means the degree to which the investigator structures the observational setting.

   Ex. A study of exploratory behavior among children in relation to empathic behavior in parents. The investigator observes mothers and children interacting. A sequence of behaviors may be observed, e.g., the approach of child to mother, response of the mother, and reaction of the child.

E. Vignettes

1. An indirect method of obtaining information to evaluate behavior
2. Based on actual situations that reflect the concepts being studied
3. The investigator assigns values to responses according to rules, to obtain a reliable and objective evaluation of the responses
4. Scoring is based on assigned values or ratings that indicate the extent to which a subject responds in relation to the "ideal" response or standard

Ex. Decision making about pharmacological pain management of postoperative patients

   a. The investigator presents a postoperative patient situation that highlights predetermined aspects of the pain experience and pharmacological pain management.
   b. Subjects communicate what they would do if they were caring for this patient and what information (cues) they used to arrive at their decisions.
   c. Cues must be identified
   d. Values must be assigned to cues
   e. Score reflects extent of use of cues in decision making

II. GUIDES FOR LOCATING MEASUREMENT INSTRUMENTS

A. Know the nature of variable to be studied
B. Consult good references on tests and measures
C. Search the periodical literature
D. Consult compiled reviews of measures
E. If no satisfactory measure is located, consider revision of an extant tool or construction of a new instrument

An excellent database of health and psychosocial instruments (HaPI) is published by the Behavioral Measurement Database Services (Perloff, 1996). The HaPI-CD permits access to 36,000 records of information on measurement instruments relevant to the health and psychosocial sciences. Available in DOS and Windows, the HaPI CD-ROM can be installed on any IBM-compatible PC with a CD-ROM drive, 640K RAM memory, and 500K free hard disk space.

III. ASSESSMENT OF VALIDITY AND RELIABILITY OF A MEASURE

A. Validity

1. Refers to whether an instrument or a test actually measures what it is supposed to measure

2. Determined by

    a. submitting the instrument to a group of judges or experts who estimate whether the *content* is representative of the universe of content of the characteristic being measured

    b. checking to see if subjects are actually engaged in the activity or are able to exhibit the quality measured by the instrument (known as *concurrent* validity, similar to *predictive* validity)

        — often presented in the form of correlational data between the measurement and the outcome or between two measures that are purported to measure the same thing

    c. studying the relationship between the theory and the measurement of the constructs, or concepts, which make up the theory (known as *construct* validity)

    d. considering the construct definition for the measure and evaluating whether the items reflect that definition (known as face or content validity)

    e. comparing the responses to those of a group already known to have a particular characteristic or behavior

B. Reliability

1. Refers to the proportion of accuracy to inaccuracy in measurement
2. Addresses the issue of stability, e.g., if a variable is measured repeatedly with the same or comparable instrument, will the same, or similar, results be obtained?
3. Determined by

    a. *test-retest*—a test is administered twice to the same subjects; if the test is reliable and the characteristic is stable, the results will be consistent

    b. *equivalent tests*—equivalent tests contain the same types of items based on the same material but the particular references and wording of items are different

        — alternate forms of a test reveal a high correlation if tests are reliable

    c. *split-half*—compares the results of one-half of the items (odd numbered) to the other half (even numbered) on a measure—

appropriate only if all the items are designed to measure the same construct

— a high correlation indicates reliability

d. *statistical tests*—yield a reliability coefficient that is obtained by applying a statistical formula to the test scores

Ex. Kuder-Richardson
Spearman Brown
Cronbach's Alpha

e. *item analysis*—a measure of internal consistency that examines the extent to which the whole test or scale is predictive of responses to individual items

— a high correlation between an item and the total score indicates the item is reliable

8

Development of
Quantitative Measures

In recent years, there has been an enormous increase in the development of quantitative measures by nursing investigators. This trend has evolved in response to the interest in studying the human behaviors and responses that are of particular interest to nurses. Although this development is not surprising since all research requires some form of observation, or measurement, the sound psychometric principles developed in earlier years by other disciplines are applicable to the activities of nursing investigators. Thus the need for valid and reliable measures with a sound theoretical foundation led to the inclusion of this chapter.

The focus of this chapter is a relatively detailed description of the process used to develop a measure of need fulfillment in the marital relationship. Increasingly, nurses have become interested in the study of social support as a construct that plays a key role in the well-being of patients. The development of the Partner Relationship Inventory (PRI) occurred as a result of that interest. The continued development of the PRI has entailed the construction of alternate forms to measure change over time, both in patients and in families.

Nurses are in a prime position to interact with clients during the course of the different phases of an illness experience. Thus they frequently can evaluate needs as they vary over time and intervene in a timely and appropriate manner. The example of the development of the PRI is offered as an encouragement to those who may wish to join the challenge of developing measures that lend themselves to capturing change as it occurs in clients and families.

I. OBJECTIVES

A. Create valid and reliable measures of behaviors and perceptions
B. Different measures according to intended populations
C. Test theory

    D.   Construct alternate forms to capture change over time

    E.   Develop culturally sensitive measures

II. METHODOLOGICAL STEPS: CONSTRUCTION OF A MEASURE

    A.   Construct a theoretical framework, based on an exhaustive review of relevant literature

        Ex. Hoskins, C. N. (1985). *The Partner Relationship Inventory.* Palo Alto, CA: Consulting Psychologists Press, Inc.

           The theoretical framework for the PRI was based on a review of literature from family theory, interpersonal conflict, and role theory. The framework is based on findings that indicate that interaction in family relationships is instrumental in fulfilling psychosocial needs of individual members. When the interaction is a true dialogue in which each participant first perceives, then complements the other's needs, the probability is greater that basic positive emotions will prevail and conflict will be minimal. Conversely, when the task of meeting specific psychosocial needs is not accomplished, conflict ensues.

    B.   Develop a construct definition

        Ex. The construct definition for the PRI is: "the perceived degree of fulfillment of interaction and emotional needs." Studies of perceptual differences in partner relationships indicate that partners who perceive that they are not receiving responses from their mates in accordance with their expectations engage in provocative, domineering, and competitive behaviors that are conducive to conflict. Other investigations support the notion that perception is of crucial importance in the immediate outcome of the interaction, as well as in the fulfillment, or lack of fulfillment, of needs.

    C.   Construct the items

        Ex. In early basic work (Mathews & Mihanovich, 1963), 400 items were constructed from an extensive review of the literature on conflict and classified into 50 problem areas distinguishing happy from unhappy relationships, 42% representing basic human needs and 36%, interaction needs. Permission was obtained to use the work in the development of the PRI.

        1.   The 50 items distinguishing happy and unhappy couples were placed in either the dimension of emotional need or interaction need, depending on content.

2. The items were classified into eight categories reflecting a specific focus, five for the interaction need dimension and three for the emotional need dimension. (A fourth dimension was omitted since a Varimax rotated factor analysis indicated it contributed to both dimensions.)

3. Each category was expanded to 10 items by formulating additional items with similar wording and essentially the same content.

4. Approximately one-half of the items were phrased in reverse form, facilitating the study of consistency in response and reduction in response set.

D. Arrange the total pool of items in a logical and smooth sequence, alternating the reverse-score items with positively phrased items

E. Construct a response format, balancing positive and negative response options

F. Submit the scale to selected experts for evaluation of items and response format by using the following criteria:

1. Do the items represent the universe of content for the construct being measured, thus reflecting content validity?
2. Are the items appropriate for the designated population?
3. Are the items situations specific?
4. Do the items contain one idea rather than multiple ideas?
5. Are person and tense consistent?
6. Are there double negatives, e.g., are negative stems combined with negatively phrased options?
7. What is the probability of response set? faking? social desirability?
8. Is the response format "balanced," e.g., an equal number of positively and negatively phrased items?
9. Are the instructions for respondents clear?
10. Do the instructions reflect whether the items are to be answered according to the moment (state) or in general (trait)?

G. Revise the scale, response format, and instructions according to the evaluations

H. Select a valid and reliable measure for the study of construct validity of the newly constructed measure

   Ex. The Marital Adjustment Test (Locke & Wallace, 1959) was selected for construct validation of the PRI.

I. Submit the newly constructed measure, the selected measure for the study of construct validity, and a demographic form to a sample of appropriate size and characteristics

J. Consider procedures to evaluate reliability, e.g., test-retest reliability requires respondents to complete the newly constructed measure at two designated times

Ex. A sample of couples completed the PRI in the morning and early evening.

K. Conduct preliminary preparation of the data

1. Evaluate missing data
2. Reverse score items as indicated
3. Calculate subscale, or category, scores for all measures as indicated

K. Estimate construct validity of the newly constructed measure

Ex. Pearson product-moment correlation coefficients were calculated between the MAT total score and each PRI category score. The validity of the PRI was demonstrated to be moderate to high (range = .40–.75). Varimax rotated factor analyses provided a useful method for determining to what degree a category enhanced the measurement of fulfillment of needs in the interaction and emotional dimensions. The factor loadings for the categories on the appropriate dimension ranged from .63–.91, thus verifying the theoretical structure of the scale.

L. Estimate reliability

Ex. Pearson product-moment correlation coefficients between total scores for the categories and constituent items verified internal consistency. Pearson product-moment correlation coefficients between responses for the morning and evening for each category supported test-retest reliability (range = .84–.95).

M. Temporal patterning

1. Nursing assessment and intervention necessitates multiple observations of behaviors over time. Qualitative and quantitative observations and measures facilitate

    a. the definition of patterns in human behavior
    b. the identification of change that occurs over time
    c. the consideration of change in relation to other behaviors or constructs

       Ex. Each of the morning and evening PRI category mean scores reflected an increase in negative feelings; however, the standard error of the difference between means for the morning and evening scores were significant for only two categories.

2. Construct alternate forms of a measure

a. A single observation of a defined behavior or interaction yields little information of value in terms of ongoing patterns within an individual or a family system. Such study necessitates a sequence of observations of behaviors, perceptions, or feelings, either directly or by a measurement scale.

Ex. The method used to develop alternate forms of the PRI included the following steps:

1. For each category the means of the 10 items from the questionnaire completed early in the day were placed in rank order of magnitude

Rank Ordering of Category 2 by Mean Values

Item	Mean
1	3.40
2	3.37
3	3.25
4	3.21
5	1.71
6	1.67
7	1.58
8	1.46
9	1.35
10	1.08

Items 1, 2, 3, and 4 are reverse-score items. The scores have not yet been reverse scored, which is reflected in the magnitude of the mean values.

2. The 10 items were divided by the serpentine method into two groupings, e.g., the items were rank ordered according to mean values in a serpentine pattern. The objectives are to

a. Equalize groups in terms of expected degree of fulfillment as reflected in responses to items
b. Achieve an approximately equal number of reverse-score items in each alternate form

Items in Category 2 Divided into Two Groups, Using the Serpentine Method

	Group		
A		B	
Item	Mean	Item	Mean
1	3.40	2	3.37
4	3.21	3	3.25
5	1.71	6	1.67
8	1.46	7	1.58
9	1.35	10	1.08
Total	11.13		10.95

3. The means of Group A were added and compared to the total of the means of Group B

4. The means were approximately equal, indicating that the alternate forms would yield comparable scores

5. The procedure was repeated for each category and for both the inventory completed early in the day and the one completed late in the day

6. The four small groups within each category, consisting of a Group A and a Group B of both the early and late forms, were examined for level of reliability

7. The group means and standard deviations were calculated, and the Pearson product-moment correlation coefficient was used to compute the group item, the interitem, and the intergroup correlation coefficients

8. The Spearman-Brown formula was used to determine the reliability levels of the groups by the split-half method

9. One alternate form of the scale was constructed by combining the five items from Group A of each of the categories into a 40-item scale. The second alternate form was constructed by combining the five items from Group B of each of the categories

References
and Bibliography

Babbie, E. (1990). *Survey research methods* (pp. 65–117). Belmont, CA: Wadsworth.

Blalock, H. (1969). *Theory construction.* Englewood Cliffs, NJ: Prentice-Hall.

Bogdan, R., & Taylor, S. (1975). *Introduction to qualitative research methods: A phenomeno-logical approach to the social sciences.* New York: Wiley.

Burns, N. (1989). Standards for qualitative research. *Nursing Science Quarterly, 2*(1), 44–52.

Burns, N., & Grove, S. K. (1993). *The practice of nursing research.* Philadelphia: W. B. Saunders.

Chenitz, W. C., & Swanson, J. (Eds.). (1986). *From practice to grounded theory: Qualitative research in nursing.* Menlo Park, CA: Addison-Wesley.

Chinn, P. L., & Jacobs, M. K. (1995). *Theory and nursing.* St. Louis, MO: C. V. Mosby.

Cohen, J. (1988). *Statistical power analysis for the behavioral sciences* (2nd ed.). Hillsdale, NJ: Erlbaum.

Crabtree, B., & Miller, W. (Eds.). (1992). *Doing qualitative research.* Newbury Park, CA: Sage.

Denzin, N., & Lincoln, Y. (Eds.). (1994). *Handbook of qualitative research.* Thousand Oaks, CA: Sage.

Devellis, R. F. (1991). *Scale development: Theory and applications.* Newbury Park, CA: Sage.

Dubin, R. (1969). *Theory building.* New York: Free Press.

Edgerton, S. (n.d.). *Guide to critique of philosophical research.* Unpublished manuscript, School of Education, New York University.

Ely, M., Anzul, M., Friedman, T., Garner, D., & Steinmetz, A. (1991). *Doing qualitative research: Circles within circles.* New York: Falmer Press.

Fink, A. (1995). *How to sample in surveys.* Thousand Oaks, CA: Sage.

Geitgey & Metz. (1973). In F. Downs & M. Newman (Eds.), *A source book of nursing research.* Philadelphia: F. A. Davis.

Giacquinta, J., Bauer, J., & Levin, J. (1993). *Beyond technology's promise.* New York: Cambridge University Press.

Given, B., & Given, C. W. (1992). Patient and family caregiver reaction to new and recurrent breast cancer. *Journal of the American Medical Women's Association, 47*(5), 201–206.

Gross, N., Giacquinta, J., & Bernstein, M. (1973). *Implementing organizational innovations.* New York: Basic Books.

Henry, G. (1990). *Practical sampling*. Thousand Oaks, CA: Sage.

Hoskins, C. N. (1980). Psychometrics in nursing research: Construction of an interpersonal conflict scale. *Research in Nursing and Health, 4,* 243–249.

Hoskins, C. N. (1988). *The Partner Relationship Inventory*. Palo Alto, CA: Consulting Psychologists Press.

Kim, J., & Mueller, C. W. (1978). *Factor analysis: Statistical methods and practical issues*. Beverly Hills, CA: Sage.

Kim, J., & Mueller, C. W. (1978). *Introduction to factor analysis: What it is and how to do it*. Beverly Hills, CA: Sage.

Kish, L. (1965). *Survey sampling*. New York: Wiley.

Light, R. J., Singer, J. D., & Willett, J. B. (1990). *By design* (pp. 186–210). Cambridge, MA: Harvard University Press.

Lincoln, Y. S., & Guba, E. G. (1985). *Naturalistic inquiry*. Beverly Hills, CA: Sage.

Locke, H. J., & Wallace, K. M. (1959). Short marital adjustment and prediction tests: Their reliability and validity. *Marriage and Family Living, 21,* 251–255.

Lofland, J., & Lofland, L. H. (1984). *Analyzing social settings: A guide to qualitative observation and analysis* (2nd ed.). Belmont, CA: Wadsworth.

Maloney, M. F. (1995). A Heideggerian hermeneutical analysis of older women's stories of being strong. *Image: Journal of Nursing Scholarship, 27*(2), 104–109.

Manchester, P. (1986). Analytic philosophy and foundational inquiry: The method. In P. Munhall & C. Oiler, *Nursing research: A qualitative perspective* (pp. 229–249). Norwalk, CT: Appleton-Century-Crofts.

Mangione, T. (1995). *Mail surveys* (pp. 38–87). Thousand Oaks, CA: Sage.

Mariano, C. (1990). Qualitative research: Instructional strategies and curricular considerations. *Nursing and Health Care, 11*(7), 354–359.

Mariano, C. (1995). The qualitative research process. In L. Talbot (Ed.), *Principles and practices of nursing research*. St. Louis, MO: C. V. Mosby.

Mathews, V. D., & Mihanovich, C. S. (1963). New orientations on marital maladjustment. *Marriage and Family Living, 25,* 300–304.

Miles, M. B., & Huberman, A. M. (1994). *Qualitative data analysis: A sourcebook of new methods*. Beverly Hills, CA: Sage.

Morse, J. (Ed.). (1991). *Qualitative nursing research: A contemporary dialogue* (Rev. ed.). Newbury Park, CA: Sage.

Munhall, P., & Boyd, C. O. (1993). *Nursing research: A qualitative perspective*. New York: National League for Nursing Press.

Northouse, L. L., Laten, D., & Reddy, P. (1995). Adjustment of women and their husbands to recurrent breast cancer. *Research in Nursing and Health, 18,* 515–524.

Nunnally, J. (1978). *Psychometric theory*. New York: McGraw-Hill.

O'Brien, M. T. (1993). Multiple sclerosis: The relationship among self-esteem, social support, and coping behavior. *Applied Nursing Research, 6*(2), 54–63.

Patton, M. (1990). *Qualitative evaluation and research methods* (2nd ed.). Newbury Park, CA: Sage Publications.

Pedhazur, E. J., & Schmelkin, L. P. (1991). *Measurement, design, and analysis: An integrated approach*. Hillsdale, NJ: Erlbaum.

Perloff, E., Director. (1996). Health and Psychosocial Instruments [CD-ROM]. Pittsburgh, PA: Behavioral Measurement Database Services.

Salant, P., & Dillman, D. (1994). *How to conduct your own survey* (pp. 53–75). New York: Wiley.

Sarter, B. (1988). *Paths to knowledge: Innovative research methods for nursing*. New York: National League for Nursing Press.

Schatzman, L., & Strauss, A. (1982). *Field research: Strategies for a natural sociology* (2nd ed.). Englewood Cliffs, NJ: Prentice-Hall.

Scott, D. W. (1983). Anxiety, critical thinking and information processing during and after breast biopsy. *Nursing Research, 32,* 24–28.

Slonim, M. (1960). *Sampling*. New York: Simon & Schuster.

Spector, P. E. (1992). *Summated rating scale construction*. Newbury Park, CA: Sage.

Strauss, A. L., & Corbin, J. (1990). *Basics of qualitative research: Grounded theory procedures and techniques*. Newbury Park, CA: Sage.

Tesch, R. (1990). *Qualitative research: Analysis types and software tools*. Bristol, PA: Falmer Press.

Waltz, C., & Bausell, R. B. (1981). *Nursing research: Design, statistics and computer analysis*. Philadelphia: F. A. Davis.

Williams, B. (1978). *A sampler on sampling*. New York: Wiley.

Appendix A

Suggested Guide
for Abstracting Research Studies

Complete bibliographic data: Include author, title, source, date, and pages.

Statement of the problem: Use direct quotes, if possible, to identify the area in which the study was conducted and purpose of the study.

Hypotheses: Use direct quotes to list hypotheses if they are presented.

Sample: Note how many subjects were in the actual sample, as well as characteristics, i.e., age level, socioeconomic status (SES), and geographic area. Note method of selecting or identifying sample.

Procedures: Outline actual steps taken in the study, i.e., sources of data, collection procedures.

Instruments: Note name(s) of instrument(s), reliability and validity of each. Summarize procedures used if new instrument was developed.

Time frame: Note time frame used in the study.

Method of analysis: Summarize statistical tests applied to the data.

Findings: Construct a concise statement of the most noteworthy findings.

Interpretations, conclusions, recommendations: Note briefly the recommendations by the author-investigator regarding application of findings and future research.

General suggestions:

1. Make notes regarding your own critique of each of the above parts, using contents of the present document.
2. Avoid the need to return to the original source.
3. Develop a hard copy or computerized filing system to speed retrieval.

Appendix B

Guide to Critique of Quantitative Research: With Examples and Practice Article

A. The Problem

1. In the introduction to the problem, what is the general problem of interest in the study?
2. Does the investigator narrow the problem area to a specific problem? If so, what is the sentence that most clearly approximates a problem statement? Evaluate the statement.
3. Does the investigator indicate the need for the study?

B. Hypotheses or Questions

1. If the study includes hypotheses, what are they? If the study does not include hypotheses, does the author indicate what questions the study is designed to answer? Evaluate each hypothesis or question.

C. Variables

1. What are the important variables in the study? Which are the independent and which are the dependent variables?

D. Definitions

1. Were the important variables defined operationally and conceptually? Evaluate the definitions.

E. Review of the Literature and Conceptual Framework

1. Does the investigator present a theoretical framework or a conceptual model from nursing? If so, what is it?
2. Can propositions be identified from review of the literature? Does the review indicate adequately what is known about the problem and variables of interest?

F. Method of Study

1. Research Approach

    a. What kind of research design was utilized?
    b. Is it appropriate for testing the hypotheses?
    c. Does the design permit control of extraneous variables? Which variables and in what way?

2. Sampling

    a. What were the actual size and characteristics of the sample?
    b. Were the criteria for sample selection indicated?
    c. What was the method of sample selection? Was it the most appropriate procedure, given the circumstances?

G. Instruments

1. What instruments were used for measurement of the variables?
2. Was the reliability of each instrument previously established? Did the investigator calculate the reliability? Were the levels adequate?
3. Was the validity of each instrument formerly established? Were the levels adequate?

H. Ethics

1. If living subjects were used in the study, did the author indicate how their rights and safety were protected? If so, were the procedures adequate?

I. Analysis of Data and Presentation of Results

1. Were the data presented in relation to each hypothesis? If not, which hypothesis, or questions, were omitted?
2. Was a summary of all the data presented? If not, what data were collected but not presented? Was a satisfactory explanation of the omission presented?
3. Were tables included? If so, was the information presented in the tables

also discussed in the text? Do the tables serve to clarify or enhance the data presentation?

4. Statistical analyses:

   a. What kinds of data were collected? (nominal, ordinal, interval, ratio?)
   b. Was a descriptive analysis of the data provided?
   c. What methods of data analyses were used? What tests of significance were used? Were the analyses appropriate to the level of data collected?

J. Interpretations and Conclusions

1. Are there statistically significant relationships supported in the study? If so, what are the relationships and are they interpreted?
2. If there are contradictions between the findings and previous research, are they discussed adequately?
3. Does the investigator relate the findings and interpretations to the framework, explaining which findings corroborate or contradict it?
4. Do the conclusions follow logically from the results?
5. Do the conclusions reflect all the results, both those that support the conceptual framework and those that do not?
6. Does the investigator relate the findings to the nursing practice? To education? To administration? Are indications for further research presented?

EXEMPLAR STUDY 1 WITH CRITIQUE

Northouse, L. L., Laten, D., & Reddy, P. (1995). Adjustment of women and their husbands to recurrent breast cancer. *Research in Nursing and Health, 18,* 515–524.

A. The Problem

Introduction

The introduction is not contained in a separate section. It appears to include the first three paragraphs of the article. In the first paragraph, the authors cite findings from studies that indicate that recurrence of cancer has implications for adjustment in both the patient and family. The studies are not, however, specific to breast cancer. The third paragraph indicates the need to study simultaneously the responses and adjustment to a recurrence of breast cancer in both the patient and family. Two purposes of the study are clearly indicated in paragraph 3, which inform the reader of the exact focus of the study, the sample to be studied, and the need for the study.

B. Hypotheses or Questions

Two research questions were posed at the end of the review of the literature:

   a. What are the differences in the levels of adjustment, support, symptom distress, hopelessness, and uncertainty reported by patients and spouses during the recurrent phase of breast cancer?
   b. What differences exist in their perceptions of the recurrence and their degree of surprise that the cancer recurred?

The research questions meet the criteria. The variables to be measured are clearly stated and sufficiently narrow as to suggest possibilities for empirical testing.
No hypotheses were stated.

C & D. Variables and Definitions

Conceptual and operational definitions are provided in the section on "Measures" for the study variables: hopelessness, social support, symptom distress, psychosocial adjustment, degree of distress related to the recurrence, and level of surprise that the cancer has returned. The variables were not treated as independent and dependent variables (see research questions).

E. Review of Related Literature

The review of the literature is a continuation of the introduction, consisting of studies of cancer patients with mixed sites. In more recent oncology studies, the confounding effect of heterogeneity of site and stage of cancer, varied treatment, and inadequate sample size have been noted. Since the authors' interest is differences between women and their spouses on the study variables at the time of recurrence of breast cancer, the literature provides scant evidence for a theoretical framework or hypotheses. There is some documentation, however, that a cancer recurrence is accompanied by increased uncertainty and worry among families; increased depression among caregivers; and increased distress, maladjustment, and symptom distress among patients. In one study (Given & Given, 1992), the psychosocial status of newly diagnosed breast cancer patients and family caregivers ($N = 21$ pairs) was compared to that of recurrent patients and caregivers ($N = 28$ pairs) over a 6-month period. More specific information is not offered.

The authors refer to a previous publication in which a preliminary model has been offered. From the text, the model is represented as including specific factors that contribute to couples' adjustments to a recurrence of breast cancer. A brief discussion of each factor, with citation of support from the literature is presented. The factors are portrayed in the following diagram.

F. Method of Study

Research Approach

The research design was not labeled. If it was exploratory, this was an appropriate design for achieving the stated purposes because the authors intended to explore a relatively new topic. Since there was a lack of empirical evidence, hypotheses were not warranted.

The design does not control for extraneous variables other than that patients were accepted into the study if they were experiencing a first-time recurrence within a time frame of 1 month and 3 years and consented to participation. One might question whether other variables contributed to the results.

Sampling

The sampling method was not identified, and no rationale or documentation for the criterion of first recurrence within a period of 1 month and 3 years was offered. The sampling method was apparently a nonrandom convenience sample

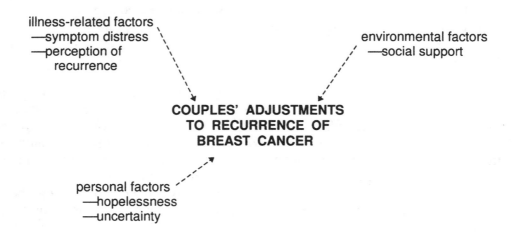

FIGURE B.1   Propositions proposed from the cited literature.

but needs to be described in greater detail, including access to subjects and sample size required to conduct the proposed analyses. One hundred and eight women and their spouses were approached, and a sample of 74 couples consented to participation, an inadequate sample size given the number of study variables (seven). The sample was relatively homogeneous in terms of ethnicity, education, employment, and family structure. Variability in other characteristics, e.g., age and time since recurrence might have been discussed in terms of possible effects on the study variables. The authors did analyze the demographic and medical data in relation to the study variables.

Instruments

In the case of all instruments, various kinds of validity were cited from previous work (refer to reprinted article for references). No information was provided on actual statistical values or characteristics of samples. Alpha coefficients were cited as established in previous work and as calculated in the present study.

The Beck Hopelessness Scale (Beck et al., 1974)
In a previous study, the alpha coefficient was reported as .93; in the present study, it was .93 and .85 for patients and spouses, respectively. The levels are acceptable.

The Mishel Uncertainty in Illness Scale (Mishel, 1981)
The alpha coefficients in the present study were acceptable at .90 and .89 for patients and spouses, respectively.

Social Support Questionnaire (Northouse et al., 1995)
The alpha coefficients in a previous study were .90 and .94 for women and their spouses, and in the present study, .87 and .86, respectively. The levels were acceptable.

The Symptom Distress Scale (McCorkle et al., 1978)
Alpha coefficients were cited for the present study only and were .84 and .85 for patients and spouses, respectively. The levels were acceptable.

Brief Symptom Inventory (Derogatis et al., 1983)
Although the measure consists of nine subscales, the overall alpha coefficient was .93 and .94 for patients and spouses, respectively. The levels were acceptable.

The Psychosocial Adjustment to Illness Scale (Derogatis et al., 1990)
The alpha levels in the present study of .90 for patients and .90 for spouses were acceptable.

H. Ethics

The procedure for protection of rights of human subjects was not described. It was stated that a consent form was signed, although the elements were not presented.

I. Analysis of Data and Presentation of Results

The authors presented the findings first for patients alone and then for spouses alone. These findings included comparisons of role problems at time of recurrence to time of initial diagnosis, and comparison of selected variables, e.g., emotional distress, to population norms (t tests of differences between means). The relationships between specific demographic variables, e.g., education, and selected main study variables, e.g., role problems, also were presented (correlation coefficients).

The patient and spouse groups also were divided into subgroups according to specific medical factors, e.g., whether receiving chemotherapy, and then examined for differences on the main study variables, e.g., role problems.

Although not all analyses were directly related to the stated research questions, they were appropriate to the data that were mainly of the interval type.

Differences between patients and spouses on the study variables as proposed in the first research question, e.g., "What are the differences in the levels of adjustment, support, symptom distress, hopelessness, and uncertainty reported by patients and spouses during the recurrent phase of breast cancer?" were presented in the text and a table. These comparisons *within* the time of recurrence yielded statistically significant differences for uncertainty, social support, and emotional distress. The measures of these variables yielded interval data, leading to the appropriate use of paired *t* tests. Both the table and text were clear.

The findings pertaining to the second research question, e.g., "What differences exist between patients and spouses in their perceptions of the recurrence and degree of surprise that the cancer returned?" were presented. They comprised the main comparisons between patients and spouses for differences between initial diagnosis and time of recurrence.

Descriptive analyses of the demographic and medical data were presented in the text.

J.   Interpretations and Conclusions

As noted previously, the scores for patients and spouses on the main study variables were compared to norms for well populations and then compared according to subgroups, e.g., whether the patient was currently in treatment. As the authors appropriately note, these findings are exploratory because the sample size in the treatment subgroups was inadequate.

The conclusions follow logically from the results with several major weaknesses: (a) the sample size(s), given the number of measures, was inadequate for drawing conclusions relative to statistical significance, (b) the kinds and levels of validity for the measures were not adequately described, and (c) the measures of which time period was most stressful and the level of surprise consisted of one item. One item is generally considered to be inadequate in terms of reliability.

Since previous work in support of the proposed relationships between variables (see diagram) appears to be very limited, the interpretation of the findings against this background was minimal.

The authors discuss the implications of the findings for practice. These implications must be regarded as highly tentative, however. The weaknesses cited previously contribute to questionable internal and external validity.

Adjustment of Women and Their Husbands to Recurrent Breast Cancer

Laurel L. Northouse, Diane Laten, and Paula Reddy

The psychosocial adjustment of women with recurrent breast cancer ($N = 81$) and their husbands ($N = 74$) were compared to determine if they report different levels of adjustment, support, symptom distress, hopelessness, and uncertainty. Women with recurrent breast cancer reported more emotional distress than their husbands, but both had a similar number of psychosocial role problems. Women and husbands differed in the amount of support and uncertainty they reported but not in the levels of symptom distress or hopelessness they perceived. Women, in contrast to their husbands, expressed more surprise that their cancer recurred and found the recurrent phase of illness more distressing than the initial diagnosis. © 1995 John Wiley & Sons, Inc.

The recurrent phase of cancer is considered one of the most difficult phases over the course of illness (McEnvoy & McCorkle, 1990; Silberfarb, Maurer, & Crouthamel, 1980; Weisman & Worden, 1986). Patients with recurrent cancer report significantly more emotional distress (Silberfarb et al., 1980), more adjustment problems (Cella, Mahon, & Donovan, 1990), and more symptom distress (Munkres, Oberst, & Hughes, 1992), than patients newly diagnosed with cancer. In one study, patients reported that the recurrence was more upsetting than the initial diagnosis, primarily because of the loss of hope they experienced when the cancer returned (Cella et al., 1990). It also has been reported that patient–professional relationships are frequently strained or ineffective during the recurrent phase of illness (Mahon, Cella, & Donovan, 1990; Wilkerson, 1991), adding to the feelings of isolation that patients experience when their cancer recurs (Wright & Dyck, 1984).

Family members also are affected by the recurrence of the cancer (Halliburton, Larson, Dibble, & Dodd, 1992). Family members report shock at the time of recurrence and increased feelings of uncertainty and worry about the ability of the patient to survive the recurrent disease (Cherkryn, 1984). In a recent study, family caregivers of patients with recurrent disease reported more depression than caregivers of patients newly diagnosed with breast cancer, due in part to the greater burden associated with providing care to patients with recurrent disease (Given & Given, 1992).

Although the recurrence of cancer affects both patients and their family members, few investigators have assessed their adjustment concurrently or compared their responses to the illness. As a result, there is little information available on whether patients and family members react to the recurrence in a similar manner or whether they have different responses to the illness—necessitating different types of interventions. The purpose of this study was to determine if differences existed in women's and husband's levels of adjustment, support, symptom distress, hopelessness, and uncertainty following the recurrence of breast cancer. A secondary purpose was to compare certain aspects of women's and husband's adjustment to the recurrence (e.g., their percep-

Laurel L. Northouse, PhD, RN, is an associate professor, and Paula Reddy, RN, BSN, is a research assistant, both at Wayne State University, College of Nursing. Diane Laten, RN, MSN, is a clinical nurse manager, St. Joseph Mercy Hospital, Ann Arbor, MI. This research was supported by an Institutional Grant to Wayne State University from the American Cancer Society.

This article was received October 4, 1994, revised, and accepted for publication on May 1, 1995.

Requests for reprints can be addressed to Dr. Northouse, Wayne State University, College of Nursing, 5557 Cass Avenue, Detroit, MI 48202.

tions of the recurrence and their degree of surprise that the cancer returned).

Several investigators have compared the responses of patients and their family members to the cancer experience (Baider & Kaplan DeNour, 1988; Cassileth et al., 1985; Clipp & George, 1992; Gotay, 1984; Northouse & Swain, 1987; Oberst & Scott, 1988). Gotay (1984) compared the problems reported by female cancer patients ($N = 73$) and their spouses ($N = 39$) and found that women with advanced disease expressed more worry about side effects of treatment and restriction of activities, while their spouses expressed more worry about their wives' emotional state and ability to survive the disease. Clipp and George (1992) also found differences in patients' and caregivers' ($N = 30$ pairs) perceptions of the illness; caregivers rated patients as having more symptoms and more fears about the future than patients themselves reported.

Some investigators have examined the amount of emotional distress that patients and family members report following the cancer diagnosis to determine if similarities or differences exist in their emotional response to the illness. Cassileth et al. (1985) assessed a heterogeneous sample of cancer patients and their relatives ($N = 201$ pairs) and found that patients reported significantly more mood disturbance than their relatives. Baider and Kaplan De-Nour (1988) found that cancer patients reported more depression than their spouses ($N = 117$ pairs), but similar levels of anxiety. Northouse and Swain (1987) found that breast cancer patients and their husbands ($N = 50$ pairs) reported similar levels of emotional distress but differed on the number of problems they had carrying out various psychosocial roles. In a longitudinal study, Oberst and Scott (1988) found different patterns of distress over time in cancer patients and their spouses ($N = 40$ couples). Spouses reported more anxiety than patients during the hospital period and 60 days later, while patients reported more anxiety than spouses just after they returned home.

Investigators have compared patients' and partners' responses during the recurrent phase of cancer in only two studies (Cherkryn, 1984; Given & Given, 1992). Chekryn conducted a small study with recurrent cancer patients and their spouses ($N = 22$ subjects) and found that couples expressed uncertainty about the future, worry about the repeated assault of the cancer, and difficulty communicating about the recurrence. Spouses, in contrast to patients, reported more concern about changes in family roles and experienced more restrictions in their leisure time activities. Given

and Given (1992) compared the psychosocial status of newly diagnosed breast cancer patients and their family caregivers ($N = 21$ pairs) and recurrent patients and their family caregivers ($N = 28$) over a 6-month period of time. The depression levels of the patients (newly diagnosed and recurrent) *decreased,* while the depression levels of their family caregivers *increased* during the 6-month period. Caregivers of patients with recurrent cancer reported the most depression of all; they reported that the recurrent cancer had a greater impact on their health and their day-to-day schedule than was reported by caregivers of the newly diagnosed group.

To date, the comparative studies of couples' adjustment to cancer indicate that both patients and spouses are affected by the cancer experience. However, previous investigators also have found that patients' and spouses' perceptions of the illness, the problems that the illness creates for them, and their emotional responses to the illness can differ at times during the course of illness. In order to assist both patients and their spouses to adjust effectively to illness, more research is needed that clarifies differences as well as similarities in their responses to illness. Based on an in-depth understanding of both partners' responses, interventions can then be tailored to address partners' individual and shared concerns.

A preliminary model, developed as a part of a larger study on couples' adjustment to recurrent cancer, was used to determine which factors were important to assess in this comparative study of couple's adjustment to recurrent cancer. The model, which was based on a review of existing literature, included personal, environmental, and illness-related factors that affect the response of both patients and husbands to breast cancer. Personal factors included the degree of hopelessness and uncertainty that partners experienced, environmental factors included the amount of social support that women and husbands perceived from one another, family, and friends, and illness-related factors included the amount of symptom distress they reported, as well as their perceptions of the recurrence and their surprise that the disease had recurred. Correlations among the major study variables have been reported previously (Northouse, Dorris, & Charron-Moore, 1995). Comparisons between women's and husbands' adjustment to recurrent breast cancer was the focus of this portion of the study.

Hopelessness has been identified as a critical factor related to adjustment, with some investigators suggesting that a collapse of hope often accompanies cancer recurrence (Cella et al., 1990).

Worden (1989) found that highly distressed patients with recurrent cancer had more pessimism and less hope for recovery. Although a few investigators have assessed patients' levels of hope, there has been no attention to spouses' levels of hope following recurrence, nor have patients' and spouses' levels of hopelessness been compared.

Uncertainty also is a key factor in couples' adjustment to cancer. Higher levels of uncertainty about the illness have been associated with poorer adjustment to cancer (Mishel, Hostetter, King, & Graham, 1984) and with more adjustment problems during radiation therapy (Christman, 1990). In a qualitative study, Chekryn (1984) found that both patients and their spouses reported increased uncertainty pertaining to the repeated assault of the cancer and to their lack of confidence in treatment plans during the recurrent phase of illness. Although uncertainty has been assessed in studies of newly diagnosed patients, further research is needed to assess both patients' and their spouses' levels of uncertainty during the recurrent phase of illness.

Social support consistently has been identified as a critical resource for patients with recurrent cancer (Spiegel, Bloom, & Gottheil, 1983; Weisman & Worden, 1986), especially in light of reports that some patients feel less support from their families and health professionals when the cancer recurs than they received initially (Cella et al., 1990; Wilkerson, 1991). Although a few investigators have examined patients' levels of support during the recurrent phase of illness, none have assessed the support perceived by spouses or family members.

Symptom distress, which is associated with either progression of the disease or aggressive treatments to control the disease, is also a key factor in adjustment to recurrent cancer (McEvoy & McCorkle, 1990). Patients with recurrent cancer report higher levels of symptom distress than newly diagnosed patients (Given & Given, 1992; Munkres et al., 1992). Furthermore, higher levels of symptom distress have been associated with increased patient dependency (Taylor, 1993), poorer patient adjustment to the recurrent cancer (Munkres et al., 1992; Worden, 1989), and added demands on family members (Halliburton, et al., 1992).

In addition to these major factors, two other factors, patients' perception of the recurrence and their degree of surprise that the cancer returned, have been identified as important. Although there are mixed reports on whether patients perceive the time of initial diagnosis or the time of recurrence as most stressful (Cella et al., 1990;

Schumacher, Dodd, & Paul, 1993; Weisman & Worden, 1986), patients' perceptions of the recurrence are related to their adjustment to the illness (Weisman & Worden, 1986). Patients' degree of surprise that the cancer has recurred also has been related to adjustment, with higher levels of surprise associated with poorer adjustment to the recurrence (Weisman & Worden, 1986). While previous investigators have identified that these two factors are important for patients' adjustment they have not been examined from the perspective of family members nor have the perceptions of patients and their family members been compared.

Based on existing research, this study was designed to address the following research questions: (a) What are the differences in the levels of adjustment, support, symptom distress, hopelessness, and uncertainty reported by patients and spouses during the recurrent phase of breast cancer? and (b) What differences exist in their perceptions of the recurrence and their degree of surprise that the cancer recurred?

METHOD

Sample

One hundred and eight women with recurrent breast cancer and their husbands were invited to participate. Of these eligible couples, 81 women (75%) and 74 husbands (68.5%) agreed to participate (74 couples). The selection criteria included women who had a first recurrence of their breast cancer, who were between 1 month and 3 years after recurrence, and who were married or living with a male partner.

The average age of the women was 53.8 (SD = 12.8, range 30–82) and the average age for men was 56.9 (SD = 12.6, range 31–81). Couples were fairly well educated, averaging 13 years of formal education for women (SD = 7.7, range 3–18) and 14 years for men (SD = 3.1, range 6–20). Approximately one third of the women and two thirds of the men were employed outside of the home. The majority of the women (96.2%) and the men (90.5%) were Caucasian. Most of the couples were in their first marriage, averaging 27 years of marriage, with no children living at home.

Approximately half (58%) of the women reported that they had a family history of breast cancer. The majority of women (84%) had a modified radical mastectomy at the time that their breast cancer was first discovered and over half

(53%) had axillary lymph node involvement at the time of initial diagnosis. The average length of time between initial diagnosis and recurrence was approximately 3 years. Most of the women were receiving some type of adjuvant treatment (88.7%), primarily hormone therapy (54%) or chemotherapy (32%), for the recurrent cancer and had known about the recurrence for an average of about 13 months. Less than one fourth of the women (18.5%) had chosen to have breast reconstruction following mastectomy.

Approximately half of the husbands (56%) reported some type of health problem of their own (e.g., hypertension, heart disease). In spite of these problems, most of the husbands (79.5%) rated their overall health as good.

Measures

Hopelessness. The Beck Hopelessness Scale (HS) was used to measure levels of hopelessness (Beck, Weissman, Lester, & Trexler, 1974). The scale consists of 20 true–false items, with higher scores indicating more hopelessness. The alpha reliability coefficient for the scale has been reported at .93 (Beck et al., 1974). In the present study, α was .85 for patients and .83 for husbands. Evidence of adequate concurrent and construct validity of the scale has been reported previously (Beck et al., 1974).

Uncertainty. The Mishel Uncertainty in Illness Scale (MUIS) was used to measure patients' levels of uncertainty (Mishel, 1981) and the Parent/Child Uncertainty Scale (PCUS) was used to measure spouses' levels of uncertainty about their wives' illness (Mishel, 1983). The MUIS consists of 34 items, while the PCUS version of the scale used with spouses consists of 31 items. In order to compare patients' and spouses' scores in the present study, three items on the patient version of the MUIS, not included in the family member version, were deleted. The questionnaires assess the amount of ambiguity, complexity, deficient information, and unpredictability that patients and their family members have about the patient's illness. Higher scores indicate more uncertainty. Adequate internal consistency and construct validity for both questionnaires have been reported previously (Mishel, 1981; Mishel, 1983; Mishel et al., 1984). In the present study the alpha reliability coefficients for the MUIS and PCUS for patients and spouses were .90 and .89.

Social Support. A modified version of the Social Support Questionnaire (SSQ), a Likert-type questionnaire, was used to measure the amount of emotional support that women and their spouses perceived from various sources (Northouse, Jeffs, Cracchiolo-Carraway, Lampman, & Dorris, 1995). Participants rated the extent to which they agreed or disagreed with 24 statements about the personal support that they perceived from three sources (spouse, family, friend); higher scores indicate more support perceived from these sources. Alpha coefficients for the SSQ were .90 for women and .94 for their spouses in a prior study (Northouse, 1988). In the present study, α was .87 for patients and .86 for husbands. Evidence of concurrent validity of the questionnaire has been reported previously (Northouse, 1988).

Symptom distress. The Symptom Distress Scale, a 13-item instrument developed by McCorkle and Young (1978), was used to measure the amount of symptom distress women experienced related to nausea, appetite, insomnia, pain, fatigue, bowel pattern, concentration, appearance, outlook, breathing, and cough. Subjects rate their degree of symptom distress on a 5-point scale with higher scores indicating more symptom distress. Breast cancer patients in this study completed the original version of the Symptom Distress Scale, while their husbands completed a modified version of the scale on which they assessed the amount of symptom distress they thought their wives were experiencing. Psychometric properties of the scale, including test–retest reliability, internal consistency, and concurrent validity of the instrument have been reported previously (McCorkle, 1987; McCorkle & Benoliel, 1983). For this study, α was .84 for patients and .85 for husbands.

Psychosocial adjustment. Two instruments were used to measure women's and husbands' levels of psychosocial adjustment: the Brief Symptom Inventory (BSI) (Derogatis & Melisaratos, 1983) and the Psychosocial Adjustment to Illness Scale (PAIS) (Morrow, Chiarello, & Derogatis, 1978).

The BSI is a 53-item measure of subjects' current emotional distress (within the past week). It consists of nine subscales: somatization, interpersonal sensitivity, obsessive compulsion, depression, anxiety, hostility, phobic anxiety, paranoid ideation, and psychotism. A total scale score is obtained by combining the number and intensity of the symptoms reported by subjects; higher scores indicate more emotional distress. Alpha coefficients for the nine dimensions ranged from .71 to .85; evidence of construct validity has been reported previously (Derogatis &

Melisaratos, 1983). In the present study, the overall α was .93 for patients and .94 for husbands.

The PAIS is a 46-item instrument used to measure subjects' psychosocial role functioning during the past month in seven domains: health care orientation, vocational environment, domestic environment, sexual relationships, extended family relations, social environment, and psychological distress. A total scale score is obtained by summing individual items within and then across the seven domains; higher scores indicate more problems carrying out various psychosocial roles. Adequate internal consistency and validity of the scale has been reported previously (Derogatis & Derogatis, 1990). In the present study, α was .90 for patients and .90 for husbands.

Additional measures. In addition to the standardized measures, information was obtained about subjects' demographic characteristics (e.g., age, education, employment status) and medical characteristics (e.g., type of surgery received, type of adjuvant treatment received, length of time since recurrence). To measure subjects' perceptions of the recurrence, they were asked to identify which period of time was most stressful for them (1 = *time of initial diagnosis*, 2 = *time of recurrence*, or 3 = *both equally stressful*). To determine subjects' degree of surprise that the cancer had recurred, they were asked to rate their level of surprise (1 = *not surprised*, 2 = *somewhat surprised*, and 3 = *very surprised*).

Procedure

The names of women eligible for the study and their spouses were obtained from medical oncology offices in the Midwest region of the United States. Couples were given two letters about the study; an introductory letter from the woman's oncologist and a brief letter describing the study from the research team. Data collection was conducted in couples' homes and informed consent was obtained.

RESULTS

Means and standard deviations for all measures are shown in Table 1. There were modest correlations between some of the independent variables, but no evidence of colinearity (see Northouse et al., 1995). The highest correlation was found between the somatization subscale of the BSI and the Symptom Distress Scale ($r = .62, p < .001$), indicating that there is some overlap between the variables. Subjects' perception of the recurrence

Table 1. Comparison of Women's and Husbands' Scores on the Major Study Variables (N = 74 Couples)

Variable	Women	Husbands	Paired t	p
Uncertainty (MUIS,[a] PCUS)				
M, SD	80.0 (16.9)	84.2 (15.7)	2.08	<.05
Range	43–148	41–121		
Hopelessness (HS)				
M, SD	3.5 (3.4)	3.8 (3.7)	.59	.56
Range	0–16	0–17		
Social support (SSQ)[b]				
M, SD	98.6 (11.3)	91.9 (10.6)	4.01	<.001
Range	73–120	69–114		
Symptom distress (SDS)				
M, SD	25.0 (8.2)	26.0 (7.9)	1.45	.15
Range	13–48	13–46		
Emotional distress (BSI)				
M, SD	.50 (.33)	.38 (.36)	2.50	<.02
Range	.02–2.3	.00–1.5		
Role adjustment (PAIS)				
M, SD	30.0 (15.8)	27.2 (16.0)	1.31	.19
Range	4–73	5–68		

[a]Scores obtained on a modified version of the MUIS. [b]Scores obtained on a modified version of the SSQ.

and their degree of surprise that the cancer recurred were not related to the independent variables.

As indicated in Table 1, the average level of emotional distress reported by women with recurrent breast cancer on the BSI was considerably higher than the level of distress (.35) reported for a normative sample of women from the general population (Derogatis, 1993). On the PAIS, the average number of psychosocial role problems reported was well above the level (16.2) reported by newly diagnosed breast cancer patients (Northouse & Swain, 1987). The descriptive data obtained on the adjustment measures indicate that women with recurrent breast cancer experience fairly high levels of emotional distress and also a considerable number of problems as they carry out their psychosocial roles.

Education was the only demographic variable that was significantly related to either of the adjustment measures, and it was related only to role adjustment (PAIS) scores, $r = -.28, p < .05$; women with less education reported more difficulty carrying out their work, family, and social roles. In regard to medical variables, there was no significant relationship between the type of surgery women had initially or the extent of their disease at the time of initial diagnosis and their scores on the adjustment measures. There also were no significant relationships between the length of time that women knew about their recurrences and their scores on the adjustment measures.

Women currently receiving treatment for their cancer reported more role problems on the PAIS than women not on treatment, $t(78) = 2.51, p < .02$. When this difference was reexamined using analysis of covariance to control for women's levels of symptom distress, women currently receiving treatment still reported significantly more role problems, $F(2,77) = 7.36, p < .01$, than women not on treatment. There was a significant difference in levels of symptom distress, $F(3,67) = 5.59, p < .01$, and the number of role problems (PAIS) reported, $F(3,67) = 4.01, p < .02$, related to treatment type. More symptom distress was reported by women who were receiving chemotherapy ($M = 27.4, SD = 8.3$) or a combination of chemotherapy and radiation therapy ($M = 34.1, SD = 7.7$) than by women receiving hormonal therapy ($M = 22.3, SD = 7.4$). More role problems also were reported by women who were receiving a combination of chemotherapy and radiation therapy ($M = 51.0, SD = 12.9$) than by women who were receiving either chemotherapy alone ($M = 33.4, SD = 16.2$) or hormonal thera-py ($M = 28.7, SD = 15.7$). These differences need to be viewed with caution, however, because the number of subjects in the various treatment categories was small.

In regard to women's perceptions of the recurrence, 40 (51.3%) reported that the time of recurrence was most stressful, 30 (38.5%) reported that the initial diagnosis was most stressful, and 8 (10.3%) said that the initial and recurrent periods were equally stressful. Adjustment did not differ as a function of the period of time women reported as most stressful. However, women who thought that the recurrent phase was most stressful were experiencing significantly more symptom distress, $t(62) = 2.08, p < .05$, than women who thought the initial phase was most stressful.

When asked how surprised they were that their cancer had recurred, 43 women (54.4%) said they were very surprised, 26 (32.9%) were somewhat surprised, and 10 (12.7%) were not surprised. BSI scores, $F(2, 74) = 5.71, p < .01$, and PAIS scores, $F(2, 74) = 3.34, p < .05$, differed for these groups. Women who were either very surprised or not at all surprised reported the most emotional distress and the most role problems following the recurrence, while women who were only somewhat surprised reported the least distress and fewer role problems.

The average level of emotional distress reported by the husbands was higher than the level (.25) reported for a normative sample of men (Derogatis, 1993) (See Table 1). The number of psychosocial role problems reported by husbands was well above the level (10.3) reported by husbands of women who were newly diagnosed with breast cancer (Northouse & Swain, 1987). Descriptive data on husbands' levels of adjustment indicated that husbands had low to moderate levels of emotional distress, but experienced considerable difficulty carrying out their various psychosocial roles.

Demographic variables were not related to husbands' scores on the adjustment measures. However, some of the medical variables, pertaining to both their wives' health and to their own health, were. For example, husbands of women who were currently on treatment reported more emotional distress than husbands of women who were not on treatment, $t(71) = 3.87, p < .001$. Husbands who had health problems of their own also reported more role adjustment difficulties than husbands who did not have health problems, $t(70) = 2.44, p < .02$. No significant relationship was found between the length of time that husbands knew about their wives' recurrence and husbands' scores on the adjustment measures.

In regard to which period of time was most stressful, 40 husbands (56%) reported that the time of initial diagnosis was the most distressing, 28 (39%) said that the time of recurrence was most distressing, and 3 (4.2%) reported that the initial and recurrent phase were equally distressing. No significant relationships were found between husbands' perceptions of the most stressful time and their scores on the adjustment measures.

When husbands were asked how surprised they were by the recurrence, 26 (36.1%) husbands said they were very surprised, 35 (48.6%) were somewhat surprised, and 11 (15.3%) were not surprised. Husbands' degree of surprise was not related to their scores on the adjustment measures.

The paired t comparisons between women's and husbands' scores on the major study variables are shown in Table 1. A significant difference was found in patients' and spouses' levels of uncertainty about the illness, with husbands reporting significantly more uncertainty than their wives. Husbands' higher uncertainty was primarily in areas related to the unpredictability and ambiguity of the illness. Women, in contrast to their husbands, reported higher levels of social support, specifically from family, $t(64) = 2.43$, $p < .02$, and friends, $t(66) = 5.71$, $p < .001$. Spouses did not differ significantly on the amount of support that they perceived from one another.

No significant difference was found between women's and husbands' levels of hopelessness; average levels of hopelessness for both were in the minimal (0–3) to mild (4–8) levels of hopelessness established by Beck et al. (1974). However, there was a wide range of scores for both women and husbands, with some subjects reporting no hopelessness and others reporting severe levels of hopelessness (scores > 15).

No significant difference was found between women's ratings of their levels of symptom distress and husbands' ratings of the amount of distress they thought their wives' were experiencing. Both women and their husbands rated fatigue as the symptom creating the most distress for women, followed by mental outlook (i.e., worry), insomnia, and pain. Women and husbands differed on their rating of concern about appearance, $t(72) = 2.71$, $p < .01$, with women reporting more distress about their appearance than their husbands thought they were experiencing. They also differed on their perceptions of intensity of the nausea, $t(72) = 2.73$, $p < .01$, the intensity of pain, $t(72) = 2.09$, $p < .04$, and the degree of insomnia, $t(72) = 2.03$, $p < .05$; husbands perceived that their wives had more difficulty with these symptoms than their wives reported.

On the adjustment measures, significant differences were found between women's and husbands' levels of emotional distress (BSI), with women reporting more distress than their husbands, primarily on subscales related to somatization $t(70) = 4.82$, $p < .001$, anxiety $t(70) = 2.55$, $p < .02$, and obsessive–compulsion (i.e., difficulty making decisions, feeling blocked in getting things done) $t(70) = 2.06$, $p < .05$. Follow-up analyses were conducted to compare women's and husbands' emotional distress scores after removing the somatization subscale (because of its moderate correlation with the Symptom Distress Scale). When the somatization subscale was removed, no significant difference was found between women's and husbands' distress scores, even though women, on average, still had higher levels of distress ($M = .45$) than their husbands ($M = .38$). On the PAIS, husbands reported as many problems carrying out their usual roles as did their wives. Their adjustment difficulties were primarily in managing domestic roles, maintaining their sexual relationship, and engaging in leisure time activities.

DISCUSSION

Differences in patients' and spouses' perceptions of the illness are apparent in these data. The majority of women were very surprised that their cancer had recurred, and a majority also reported that the period of time surrounding their recurrence was more stressful than the time when their cancer was first diagnosed. The majority of husbands, on the other hand, were only somewhat surprised by the recurrence and perceived the time of initial diagnosis as more stressful than the time of the recurrence. One explanation may be that women and men view the course of breast cancer differently at the outset. Perhaps women see breast cancer as a disease that can be treated successfully and in most cases cured, while their husbands see breast cancer in a more ominous light, as a life-threatening disease that has the likelihood of returning. Hence, the initial diagnosis is more of a concern to husbands, while the recurrence of the cancer is more of a surprise and concern for women.

A curvilinear relationship was found between surprise and women's adjustment scores, with women who reported being only somewhat surprised having the least emotional distress and role problems. Other investigators have examined the issue of surprise and patients' adjustment to recurrent cancer and the findings vary. Weisman and Worden (1986) found a positive linear relationship between surprise and emotional distress, while Cella et al. (1990) found no relationship between surprise and adjustment, but did find a curvilinear relationship between surprise and intrusive stress response (e.g., heightened arousal, intrusive dreams, vulnerability). Patients who hold the moderate position may fare better because they have a more realistic appraisal of their illness; they are neither overly pessimistic nor overly optimistic. Furthermore, because of their somewhat guarded position, they are less likely to be thrown off balance when the cancer recurs.

Significant differences were found between patients' and spouses' levels of uncertainty about the illness, support, and emotional distress. On the other hand, no significant differences emerged in the number of role problems they experienced nor in the amount of hopelessness or symptom distress they reported. Although women reported more emotional distress than their husbands, when the somatization subscale was removed from the comparison no significant difference was found; this indicates that most of the difference in their overall distress was due to the greater number of somatic symptoms reported by women versus their husbands on the emotional distress measure (BSI).

Both women and their husbands reported a sizable number of problems carrying out their various psychosocial roles after the cancer returned; this number was nearly twice that reported by newly diagnosed breast cancer patients and their husbands (Northouse & Swain, 1987). The increase in role problems for women was due in part to the symptom distress they were experiencing as a result of the treatments used to arrest the progression of the disease. Husbands' role difficulties were evidently primarily in sexual and social role (leisure time) areas. Given the reciprocal relationship that has been reported between the role problems of cancer patients with recurrent disease and their partners (Northouse et al., 1995), it is possible that, as women's role problems increased, so did their husbands'; husbands altered their roles (i.e., decreased leisure activities) to compensate for their wives' difficulties. Those husbands who had their own health problems faced the added difficulty of trying to manage their role limitations at the same time they needed to assist their wives.

Although both patients' and spouses' levels of uncertainty were comparable to the levels reported by other cancer patients (Mishel & Epstein, 1990), it is noteworthy that spouses in this study reported more uncertainty than their wives. Spouses were troubled by the changing course of their wives' illness, the lack of clarity about what would be happening next, and their inability to predict how long the illness would last or how much distress their wives may experience on a day-to-day basis. Overall, the findings indicate that spouses lacked a framework for understanding the nature and course of their wives' recurrent cancer. Spouses may have more uncertainty because they have less contact with health professionals and, therefore, have fewer opportunities to get information directly. A number of investigators have reported on the difficulties that family members of cancer patients have in obtaining information from professionals (Northouse & Northouse, 1987; Oberst & James, 1985; Wilson & Morse, 1991). The findings of this study and others suggest that health professionals need to develop interventions to ensure that spouses have direct access to information about the nature and expected course of their wives' illness. It is not sufficient to assume that spouses will get all the information they need from their wives. Spouses have legitimate needs for information and may adjust more effectively to the illness when they receive it.

Breast cancer patients in this study perceived more support than their husbands. Perhaps this is not surprising, since the women had higher levels of emotional distress and, therefore, may have needed more support. However, husbands were experiencing a fair number of role problems and also reported more uncertainty about the illness than their wives, suggesting that they also had needs for support. Perhaps husbands perceived less support because family and friends directed their supportive energies primarily toward the patient rather than them, a finding reported in other studies of cancer patients and their family members (Northouse, 1988; Oberst & James, 1985). It is also possible that husbands, as men, have fewer sources of support than women. Hence, husbands' lower levels of support may be related more to the issue of gender than to their needs for support.

No significant differences were found between the levels of hopelessness reported by women and their husbands. On the average, patients and husbands reported levels of hopelessness in the minimal to mild range, suggesting that they were able to maintain fairly hopeful outlooks about their futures despite the advanced stage of the cancer. However, there was a subgroup patients and a subgroup of husbands who had very high levels of hopelessness. Not only did these patients and husbands have a very poor outlook about their future, but they also experienced higher levels of emotional distress and role problems (Northouse et al., in press) suggesting that they would benefit from interventions by health professionals.

There were also no significant differences between patients' and spouses' reports of symptom distress. For the most part, husbands were fairly accurate in their assessments of their wives' *overall* level of symptom distress, even though they rated some of the individual symptoms (i.e., appearance, insomnia) differently. Typically, when differences on individual items appeared, husbands rated their wives as having more symptoms than their wives reported, a finding also reported by Clipp and George (1992) in their study of cancer patients and their caregivers. The fact that both patients and their husbands found fatigue as the symptom causing the most difficulty suggests that symptom management related to fatigue is an important area that health professionals need to address.

The results point to specific areas that need further investigation. First, longitudinal studies are needed to assess similarities and differences in partners' adjustment over time. Oberst and Scott (1988) and Given and Given (1992) have started to document differences in patients' and spouses' patterns of adjustment, but more research is necessary in order to determine *what* type of assistance each partner needs and *when* it should be provided. Second, there is a need for studies of the nature of spouses' uncertainty regarding their wives' illness to determine which factors affect spouses' uncertainty (e.g., limited professional contact) and what strategies can be used to reduce it. Third, studies are needed to identify couples at greater risk of poorer adjustment to recurrent illness. Hopelessness appears to be one factor that places both patients and their husbands at risk of more adjustment difficulties during the recurrent phase of illness (Northouse et al., 1995) and warrants further investigation.

Overall, the findings suggest that there are similarities and differences in partner's responses to recurrent cancer; partners' responses are not simply a mirror image of one another. Similarities were evident in women's and husbands' role problems, levels of hopelessness, and assessment of symptom distress. Differences, on the other hand, were evident in their perceptions of the recurrent illness, their levels of uncertainty, and the degree of support they perceived from family and friends. The results suggest that health professionals need to conduct psychosocial assessments with both women and their partners in order to gain a better understanding of each person's response to the illness. Intervention strategies will be more effective when health professionals take into consideration each partner's unique response as well as their shared responses to the illness.

REFERENCES

Baider, L.A., & Kaplan De-Nour, A. (1988). Adjustment to cancer: Who is the patient—The husband or the wife? *Israel Journal of Medical Sciences, 24,* 631–636.

Beck, A.T., Weissman, A., Lester, D., & Trexler, L. (1974). The measurement of pessimism: The hopelessness scale. *Journal of Consulting and Clinical Psychology, 42,* 861–865.

Cassileth, B.R., Lusk, E.J., Strouse, T.B., Miller, D.S., Brown, L.L., & Cross, P.A. (1985). A psychological analysis of cancer patients and their next-of-kin. *Cancer, 55,* 72–76.

Cella, D.F., Mahon, S.M., & Donovan, M.I. (1990). Cancer recurrence as a traumatic event. *Behavioral Medicine, 16,* 15–22.

Cherkryn, J. (1984). Cancer recurrence: Personal meaning, communication, and marital adjustment. *Cancer Nursing, 7,* 491–498.

Christman, N.J. (1990). Uncertainty and adjustment during radiotherapy. *Nursing Research, 39,* 17–20.

Clipp, E.C., & George, L.K. (1992). Patients with cancer and their spouse caregivers. *Cancer, 69,* 1074–1079.

Derogatis, L.R. (1993). *The Brief Symptom Inventory (BSI): Administration, scoring and procedures manual* (3rd ed.). Minneapolis: National Computer Systems.

Derogatis, L.R., & Derogatis, M.F. (1990). *The Psychosocial Adjustment to Illness Scale: Administration, scoring and procedures manual—II.* Towson, MD: Clinical Psychometric Research.

Derogatis, L.R., & Melisaratos, N. (1983). The Brief Symptom Inventory: An introductory report. *Psychological Medicine, 13,* 595–605.

Given, B., & Given, C.W. (1992). Patient and family caregiver reaction to new and recurrent breast cancer. *Journal of the American Medical Women's Association, 47,* 201–206.

Gotay, C.C. (1984). The experience of cancer during early and advanced stages: The view of patients and their mates. *Social Science and Medicine, 18,* 605–613.

Halliburton, P., Larson, P.J., Dibble, S., & Dodd, M.J. (1992). The recurrent experience: Family concerns during cancer chemotherapy. *Journal of Clinical Nursing, 1,* 275–281.

Mahon, S., Cella, D., & Donovan, M. (1990). Psychosocial adjustment to recurrent cancer. *Oncology Nursing Forum, 17 (Suppl.)*, 47–52.

McCorkle, R. (1987). The measurement of symptom distress. *Seminars in Oncology Nursing, 3*, 248–256.

McCorkle, R., & Benoliel, J.Q. (1983). Symptom distress, current concerns, and mood disturbances after diagnosis of life-threatening disease. *Social Science and Medicine, 17*, 431–438.

McCorkle, R., & Young, K. (1978). Development of a symptom distress scale. *Cancer Nursing, 1*, 373–387.

McEnvoy, M.D., & McCorkle, R. (1990). Quality of life issues in patients with disseminated breast cancer. *Cancer, 66*, 1416–1421.

Mishel, M. (1981). The measurement of uncertainty in illness. *Nursing Research, 30*, 258–263.

Mishel, M. (1983). Parents' perception of uncertainty concerning their hospitalized child. *Nursing Research, 32*, 324–330.

Mishel, M., & Epstein, D. (1990). *Uncertainty in Illness Scales manual*. Tucson: College of Nursing, University of Arizona.

Mishel, M.H., Hostetter, T., King, B., & Graham, V. (1984). Predictors of psychosocial adjustment in patients newly diagnosed with gynecological cancer. *Cancer Nursing, 7*, 291–299.

Morrow, G.R., Chiarello, R.J., & Derogatis, L.R. (1978). A new scale for assessing patients' psychosocial adjustment to medical illness. *Psychological Medicine, 8*, 605–610.

Munkres, A., Oberst, M.T., & Hughes, S. (1992). Appraisal of illness, symptom distress, and mood states in patients receiving chemotherapy for initial and recurrent disease. *Oncology Nursing Forum, 19*, 1201–1209.

Northouse, L.L. (1988). Social support in patients' and spouses' adjustment to breast cancer. *Nursing Research, 37*, 91–95.

Northouse, L.L., Dorris, G., & Charron-Moore, C. (1995). Factors affecting couples' adjustment to recurrent breast cancer. *Social Science and Medicine, 41*, 69–76.

Northouse, L.L., Jeffs, M., Cracchiolo-Carraway, A., Lampman, L., & Dorris, G. (1995). The emotional distress reported by women and husbands prior to a breast biopsy. *Nursing Research, 44*, 196–201.

Northouse, P.G., & Northouse, L.L. (1987). Communication and cancer: Issues confronting patients, health professionals and family members. *Journal of Psychosocial Oncology, 5*, 17–46.

Northouse, L.L., & Swain, M.A. (1987). Adjustment of patients and husbands to the initial impact of breast cancer. *Nursing Research, 36*, 221–225.

Oberst, M.T., & James, R.H. (1985). Going home: Patient and spouse adjustment following cancer surgery. *Topics in Clinical Nursing, 7(1)*, 46–57.

Oberst, M.T., & Scott, D. (1988). Postdischarge distress in surgically treated cancer patients and their spouses. *Research in Nursing & Health, 11*, 223–233.

Schumacher, K.L., Dodd, M.J., & Paul, S.M. (1993). The stress process in family caregivers of persons receiving chemotherapy. *Research in Nursing & Health, 16*, 395–404.

Silberfarb, P.M., Mauer, H., & Crouthamel, C. (1980). Psychosocial aspects of neoplastic disease: I. Functional status of breast cancer patients during different treatment regimens. *American Journal of Psychiatry, 137*, 450–455.

Spiegel, D., Bloom, J.R., & Gottheil, E. (1983). Family environment as a predictor of adjustment to metastatic breast carcinoma. *Journal of Psychosocial Oncology, 1*, 33–43.

Taylor, E.J. (1993). Factors associated with meaning in life among people with recurrent cancer. *Oncology Nursing Forum, 20*, 1399–1405.

Weisman, A., & Worden, J.A. (1986). The emotional impact of recurrent cancer. *Journal of Psychosocial Oncology, 3*, 5–15.

Wilkerson, S. (1991). Factors which influence how nurses communicate with cancer patients. *Journal of Advanced Nursing, 16*, 677–688.

Wilson, S., & Morse, J.M. (1991). Living with a wife undergoing chemotherapy. *Image, 23*, 78–84.

Worden, J.W. (1989). The experience of recurrent cancer. *CA—A Cancer Journal for Clinicians, 39*, 305–310.

Wright, K., & Dyck, S. (1984). Expressed concerns of adult cancer patient's family members. *Cancer Nursing, 7*, 371–374.

EXEMPLAR STUDY 2 WITH CRITIQUE

Scott, D. W. (1983). Anxiety, critical thinking and information processing during and after breast biopsy. *Nursing Research, 32,* 24–28.

A. The Problem

The introduction (para. 1) is concise and clear, and provides a brief but appropriate indication of the need for the study. Scott might have elaborated further on the need by addressing the behaviors to be studied and the implications for the nursing practice.

   Although the research question is not posed in question form as a possible relationship between variables, it is clearly indicated in para. 2. "The goals of the study were to determine relations among . . . three variables of during and after acute life crisis and to examine how they change over time in a group of women facing a breast biopsy for possible cancer diagnosis."

   The statement was provided early in the report so that the reader will know the exact focus of the study and the sample on which the study will be done.

B. Hypotheses

The underlying assumption of the hypotheses is that patients who undergo a breast biopsy are under stress. The way in which the individual copes with that stress is viewed from the theoretical perspective of Lazarus (source is given in reprinted article). Lazarus proposes two dimensions of coping, e.g., cognitive performance and regulation of emotion.

Hypothesis 1
H_1 states: "There will be a positive relationship between level of state anxiety and judged duration during crisis and six to eight weeks post-crisis."

Hypothesis 2
H_2 states: "There will be a negative relationship between level of state anxiety and critical thinking ability during crisis and six to eight weeks post-crisis."

Hypothesis 3
H_3 states: "There will be a negative relationship between critical thinking ability and judged duration during crisis and six to eight weeks post-crisis."

Hypothesis 4

H_4 states: "The combination of state anxiety level and critical thinking ability is a better predictor of variance in judged duration than is either state anxiety or critical thinking taken separately during crisis and six to eight weeks post-crisis."

Hypotheses 5–7

H_5 states: "State anxiety level will be higher during crisis than at six to eight weeks post-crisis."

H_6 states: "Critical thinking ability will be lower during crisis than at six to eight weeks post-crisis."

H_7 states: "Judged duration will be greater during crisis than at six to eight weeks post-crisis."

C. Variables

The variables to be measured were anxiety level, critical thinking ability, and capacity to process information. They were clearly stated and sufficiently narrow as to suggest possibilities for empirical testing. In H_3, critical thinking ability is treated as a dependent variable rather than an independent variable as in H_2 and H_4.

D. Definitions

While no separate section on definitions was provided, they were incorporated in the section on "Method." Both conceptual and operational definitions were provided for *anxiety* (para. 15), *critical thinking ability* (para. 16), and *capacity to process information*, as indicated by judged duration of time (para. 17).

E. Review of the Literature and Conceptual Framework

The review of the literature draws primarily on the theory and work of Lazarus and Lazarus & Averill. Although the work of Beier is cited as support for that of Lazarus, the complexity and directionality of the hypotheses require a more in-depth review. The works pertaining to time estimation as an indicator of cognitive performance also are limited, with inadequate citation of essential aspects of the studies.

Scott synthesizes the review of the literature in the final paragraphs (paras. 9–11), drawing upon the theory by Lazarus and the conclusions drawn by authors of cited studies. Although the imposed limitations of space for the literature review in a periodical require consideration, the complexity of deriving hypotheses from the propositions needs more explication.

A suggested diagram of axiomatic propositions from the cited literature is offered next.

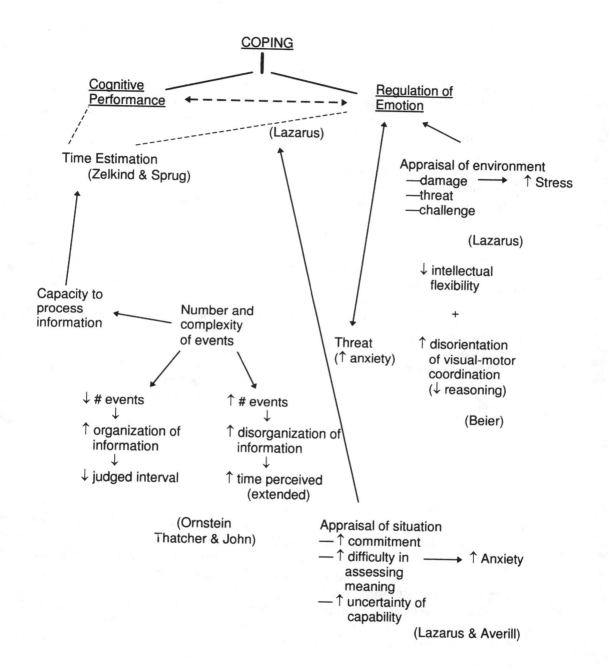

FIGURE B.2   Axiomatic propositions from the cited literature. Response to stress.

H_1 is derived from the proposition that proposes a relationship between time estimation (the cognitive aspect of coping) and anxiety (the affective component of coping). A direct relationship is evident in the diagram.

In the translation of the proposition into a testable hypothesis, "judged duration" will need to be accepted by the reader as an index of "information processing" ability, which, in turn, is viewed as the dimension of coping known as cognitive performance. Coping (according to Lazarus) embodies the two dimensions that are thought by theorists to be interactive and complex, sometimes in an indirect manner.

There is no cited literature that supports or refutes the nature of the proposed relationship during 6 to 8 weeks postcrisis. The reader might wonder why at the time of supposed resolution, the relationship might not be changed in some way.

H_2 appears to be derived from the work of Beier. The reader again needs to accept, however, the translation of the proposition to the hypothesis, as well as the conclusions drawn by Beier. Specifically, is critical thinking ability an index of intellectual flexibility + reasoning ability, which, in turn, are intended as indices of cognitive performance?

The support for H_3 is not evident in the review of the literature (as may be determined from the diagram).

H_4 combines the proposed relationships in H_1–H_3.

Although there are no cited studies to support H_5–H_7, they would be appropriate as research questions. It might have been well to assess the differences in levels of the three variables between the two times of testing and omit the second parts of H_1, H_2, and H_3.

F. Method of Study

Research Approach

The research design was labeled as exploratory, an appropriate design for testing the hypotheses. The design also could be labeled correlational. When the empirical evidence is insufficient to warrant directional hypotheses, nondirectional hypotheses—or ancillary research questions—often are proposed. Without a more in-depth review of the literature, this judgment cannot be conclusively made by the reader of the article.

The design does not control for extraneous variables other than that patients were accepted into the study if they were able to participate, afebrile, and had no previous diagnosis of cancer. One might question whether variables other than the designated predictors contributed to the results.

Sample

Eighty-five women admitted for a surgical biopsy comprised the sample. The sample characteristics are cited. Only subjects subsequently found to have a benign lesion were included and retested in the postcrisis time. No rationale or documentation for imposing the criteria for inclusion or exclusion were offered.

The sampling method was apparently a nonrandom convenience sample. The exact sampling procedure needs to be described in greater detail, including access to subjects, information that was provided to potential participants, and sample size required to test the hypotheses with documentation.

Such issues as the wide variability in the demographic characteristics, e.g., age and education, need to be discussed from the perspective of possible effect on the criterion variable ("information processing," considered to be an index of coping). If the sample was voluntary, but drawn according to specified characteristics to serve as a control, this needs to be discussed. Other possible sources of extraneous variance should be noted.

G. Instruments

The State-Trait Anxiety Inventory (Spielberger et al.)

The Anxiety-State Scale
—defined as transitory anxiety
    The reported reliabilities are variable and lack clarity. The reported validity is not clear in terms of kind, level, and standardization sample.

The Anxiety-Trait Scale
—defined as disposition to stressful situations with varying levels of anxiety intensity; the degree to which stimuli are perceived as threatening
    The reliability is not reported for the scale. The cited correlation coefficients with other standard trait anxiety measures are good; standardization samples are not specified.

The Watson Glaser Critical Thinking Appraisal (CTA)
—defined as an aspect of the general reasoning and problem-solving process necessary for the interpretation of information, formation of judgments, and decision making
    The reported reliability is adequate. The cited construct validity has a wide range. The standardization sample is not specified.

Judged Duration
—defined as the estimation of time required to complete the CTA
    The measurement procedure was developed by Scott. Reliability and validity issues were not addressed.

H. Ethics

The procedure for protection of rights of human subjects requires discussion.

I.   Analysis of Data and Presentation of Results

H_1–H_3 were tested by the Pearson product-moment correlation coefficient, H_4 by multiple regression, and H_5–H_7 by the t test for correlated means, all appropriate statistics for the interval data that were collected. The second part of H_1 and H_4 were confirmed, e.g., the proposed relationships for time of postcrisis. Both H_5 and H_6 were confirmed, e.g., state anxiety was higher and critical thinking was lower during crisis than at the postcrisis time. H_7 was not confirmed. The data for the main study variables were of the interval type; thus the statistical analyses and tests of significance were appropriate. The findings were presented in one table, which served to reinforce the text presentation.

Descriptive statistics for the study variables were presented in table form but not for demographic and medical data. Although the table enhanced the presentation, other descriptive statistics should be presented.

J.   Interpretations and Conclusions

Scott begins the discussion by addressing the ability to estimate time and how it was proposed to be compromised under conditions of stress. The discussion of this highly complex construct was appropriate, as was the issue of its measurement.

The finding of no relationship between anxiety and critical thinking was contrary to the results of previous research. Scott provides a good discussion, including the nature of a curvilinear, rather than a linear, relationship.

Similarly, Scott suggests plausible reasons as to why the proposed positive relationship between critical thinking ability and judged duration was not confirmed.

Finally, the variation in the level of variable measures from the initial time to the postcrisis time was in the predicted direction, a noteworthy finding.

Scott presents an excellent discussion in the section on "Conclusions," to which the reader is referred. The conclusions follow logically from all results. Scott recognized that application to practice is premature. Instead, appropriate questions are raised and suggestions for further studies are made.

Anxiety, Critical Thinking and Information Processing During and After Breast Biopsy

DIANE W. SCOTT

State anxiety (STAI), critical thinking ability (CTA), and judged duration were tested for coping relatedness and change over time in 85 women, aged 18 to 60, who were experiencing breast biopsy. Participants were tested after hospital admission but before diagnostic results were known. Six to eight weeks later, women whose results were benign were tested again—when an acute crisis is considered concluded. Findings revealed extremely high state anxiety levels prior to biopsy and compromised reasoning ability at a critical time when demands on cognitive functioning were high.

For a woman, hospitalization for breast biopsy is a time of life crisis. Over 110,000 women are diagnosed with breast cancer each year; about 37,000 others die of the disease (American Cancer Society, 1980). Many more consult physicians with suspicious lumps or thickenings. In fact, 25 percent of physician visits by women are concerned with an abnormal finding in the breast (Townsend, 1980).

In order to contribute further knowledge about how people cope with stress, an exploratory study was undertaken to examine the three variables of anxiety level, critical thinking ability, and capacity to process information (time perception) found important to coping response. The goals of the study were to determine relations among these three variables during and after acute life crisis and to examine how they change over time in a group of women facing a breast biopsy for possible cancer diagnosis.

The Literature

Response to stress is a coping operation with a dual function: problem-solving and regulation of emotion (Lazarus, 1978). The process embodies both cognitive and affective domains, which many theorists believe to be related. The interaction between the two variables is complex and, at times, indirect.

Cognitive performance and anxiety level have been most clearly and significantly related in those studies that have: (1) specified type of anxiety (state and trait) (Meyers and Martin, 1974; Tennyson and Woolley, 1971; Tennyson and Boutwell, 1973); (2) recognized a curvilinear relationship between anxiety level and cognitive performance (Moon and Lair, 1970); and (3) differentiated between levels of anxiety (Mazzai and Goulet, 1969; Mandler and Sarason, 1952; O'Neill, 1972) and general approach to problem-solving (Beier, 1951; Martindale and Greenough, 1973). Those studies concerned with test anxiety have come closest to real life and in the main show that anxiety and performance are related (Sarason, 1972).

Beier (1951) illustrated the relationship between reasoning ability and anxiety when he found that loss of intellectual flexibility and a disorientation of visual-motor coordination occurred when subjects were faced with threat. He concluded that in real-life circumstances, anxiety increases when threat places a strain on normal coping strategies, intensified by an increased belief in one's inability to cope. Lazarus and Averill (1972) contended that anxiety and cognitive appraisal of the situation are mutually dependent. The level of anxiety increases when a set of circumstances involves heavy commitment, produces difficulty with the assessment of meaning or structure, and includes uncertainty about coping ability. Level of anxiety, then, reflects tension created by reduced cognitive ability to symbolize, structure, organize, or to assign full meaning to an event.

Time perception, more specifically the human estimation of an interval of time, correlates with both emotion and cognitive functioning. In over 2,000 studies concerned with time estimation and the experience of duration, results have been inconclusive and difficult to interpret due to the (1) variety of measurement methods, (2) differences in length and content of the time interval, (3) variability of experimental conditions employed, and (4)

Accepted for publication April 12, 1982.
This study was supported in part by Research Facilitation Grant NU 00596, DHEW.

DIANE W. SCOTT, PH.D., R.N., is a nurse scientist at Memorial Sloan-Kettering Cancer Center, New York City.

diversity in interpretation of results (Zelkind and Sprug, 1974).

Recent studies have not conclusively clarified the behavioral meaning of human time perception but offer an interpretation. The cognitive view expresses time perception as a function of the individual's capacity to process information. This capacity is influenced by the number and complexity of events construed by the individual. Ornstein (1969) defines the process describing people as having an "intake register" and a "storage space" when it comes to incorporating and operating on information in the environment. A given period of time is said to be perceived as extended or lengthened if the number of events taken in by the register is increased and the information is stored in a disorganized fashion. Conversely, the interval is reduced when the number of events entering the system is decreased or the person is better able to organize, chunk, or code the information.

Ornstein's conclusions have been supported by the work of Thatcher and John (1977). Their research interprets time perception as a function of the cytoarchitecture of the cerebral cortex and its neurochemical linkages with sensory input. According to their findings, a neural representational system in the brain increases and decreases in size according to the amount of information loaded into it. As the spatial size of neurological structures increases, the more complex the individual's experience or the greater amount of information taken in. Thatcher and John (1977) and Ornstein (1969) contend that the size of these structures is related to a person's reconstruction of an interval of time.

Stress occurs when an individual construes environmental stimuli as damaging, threatening, or challenging (Lazarus, 1978). During hospitalization and the possibility of life-threatening diagnosis, the number and rate of presentation of stimuli are increased substantially from normal. The newness of the experience is a major factor.

The patient admitted into such circumstances has busy "intake register"; one that fast becomes overloaded. The individual must organize and draw meaning from the rapidly presented information and use mental operations (memory and problem solving) to make sound decisions important to future survival. Thus, storage space may become disorganized and overloaded.

When an individual is under stress, anxiety level is expected to be elevated, general reasoning ability reduced, and the capacity to process information depressed. In addition, research results have correlated anxiety levels, cognitive performance, and time perception. These were anticipated to be related on both testing occasions. Predictions about the nature of the relationship of variables and changes in their levels given two intensities of stress formed the basis for hypotheses formation.

The Hypotheses

I. There will be a positive relationship between level of state anxiety and judged duration during crisis and six to eight weeks post-crisis.
II. There will be a negative relationship between level of state anxiety and critical thinking ability during crisis and six to eight weeks post-crisis.
III. There will be a negative relationship between critical thinking ability and judged duration during crisis and six to eight weeks post-crisis.
IV. The combination of state anxiety level and critical thinking ability is a better predictor of variance of judged duration than is either state anxiety or critical thinking taken separately during crisis and six to eight weeks post-crisis.
V. State anxiety level will be higher during crisis than at six to eight weeks post-crisis.
VI. Critical thinking ability will be lower during crisis than at six to eight weeks post-crisis.
VII. Judged duration will be greater during crisis than at six to eight weeks post-crisis.

Method

Eighty-five women admitted to a large, urban cancer center for surgical biopsy to ascertain presence of carcinoma of the breast were included in the study. Subjects were between the ages of 18 and 60, with educational levels ranging from high school through college; socioeconomic levels ranging from 1 through 6 according to the Hamburger classification (1957). Subjects voluntarily consented to take part in the study and were able to participate in and tolerate the testing procedures. No subject had a previous diagnosis of cancer and all were afebrile on both testing occasions.

The biopsy procedure was surgical, performed with subjects under general anesthesia. Only subjects subsequently found to have benign conditions were included and retested in the post-crisis period, six to eight weeks later (calculated from date of biospy procedure).

Anxiety was measured by the State-Trait Anxiety Inventory (STAI) (Spielberger, Gorsuch, and Lushene, 1970), consisting of two 20-item instruments designed to measure state and trait aspects of anxiety. The A-state scale measures how the subject feels at a particular moment in time, indicating a level of transitory anxiety characterized by feelings of apprehension and tension and autonomic-nervous-system-induced symptoms. The characteristics assessed by the A-state scale include feelings of tension, nervousness, worry, and apprehension. (Reliability range .16 to .54; alpha coefficient range .83 to .92, typically higher under stress; construct validity, point biserial range .60 to .73; alpha range .83 to .94). The A-trait scale measures disposition to respond to stressful situations with varying levels of A-state intensity and the degree to which presenting stimuli are perceived as dangerous or threatening. It elicits data on the subject's general level of arousal and is predictive of anxiety proneness. Correlations with other standard trait anxiety instruments have been well-established: IPAT Anxiety Scale (.75 to .77); Taylor Manifest Anxiety Scale (.79 to .83); and Affect Adjective Checklist (.51 to .52). Construct validity has been determined by subjecting participants to testing under stress and nonstress conditions. Scores across conditions are shown to increase as the experimental stress conditions become more intense. Both scale segments are shown to have high degrees of internal consistency (Spielberger, Gorsuch, and Lushene, 1970).

Critical thinking ability was determined by the Watson-Glaser Critical Thinking Appraisal (CTA) (Watson and Glaser, 1964), an instrument designed to measure the general reasoning process used on a daily basis, as an individual works, reads a newspaper or magazine and participates in discussions and conversation. Critical thinking is an aspect of the general reasoning and problem-solving processes necessary for the interpretation of information, formation of judgments and decision-making in everyday life. The test consists of 100 items divided into five subcategories of thinking important to one's overall ability at critical appraisal. The subcategories are: inference, recognition of assumptions, deduction, interpretation, and evaluation of arguments (reliability, .77 to .87; construct validity, .34 to .75) (Watson and Glaser, 1964).

The capacity to process information was measured by time estimation, in this case, judged duration (Ornstein, 1969; Thatcher and John, 1977). Judged duration is a verbal estimate of a previously experienced duration interval as compared to actual or clock time (reliability, .62 to .84) (Doob, 1971). The interval in this study was the time taken to complete the Watson-Glaser CTA. Response was requested in minutes, then compared to a standard (clock or actual time) as measured by a subject-controlled electronic timer with remote control. Calculation of judged duration is as follows:

$$JD = \frac{T_j - T_a}{T_a} \times 100$$

Where, JD = judged duration
T_j = judged time
T_a = actual or clock time

Judged duration is the error or difference, expressed as a percent, between a subjective judgment of time and the objective length of the interval (clock time). Participants were tested on two occasions—once following hospital admission, but before biopsy and knowledge of diagnostic results; and six to eight weeks after the individual had been notified that results of the breast biopsy indicated a nonmalignant condition. The six to eight weeks period is when an acute crisis is considered to be resolved or concluded (Bloom, 1963; Lewis, Gottesman and Gutstein, 1979). An informed consent form stating the purpose of the study, nature of subject participation, safety and liability factors, confidentiality and agreement concerning freedom to withdraw at any time was signed by each subject prior to testing. Oral temperature was taken with an IVAC digital thermometer to control for the documented effect on increased body temperature on time perception (Baddeley, 1966; Eson and Kafka, 1952; Hoagland, 1933, 1966; and Pfaff, 1968). Following an initial interview for collection of socio-demographic data, test instruments were administered in the following order: STAI, CTA (YM and ZM forms used during the two testing sessions and alternately in the sample to control for sequence

effect), JD. At the start and end of the CTA, subjects pressed a button activating an electronic timer with remote control. Testing was not time-limited. Immediately following deactivation of the timer, subjects were asked for a verbal estimation of elapsed time. Actual time was obtained from the timer's digital read-out.

Retesting repeated the same protocol and took place six to eight weeks following biopsy at a location convenient for the subject, most often her home. Subjects were debriefed following the second testing session.

Results

Relations between pairs of variables were tested using the Pearson product-moment correlation coefficient (Table 1).

Hypothesis I, predicting a positive relationship between level of state anxiety and judged duration, was confirmed at the six-week post-biopsy testing, but no correlation was found at the time of acute crisis.

Hypothesis II, predicting a negative relationship between state anxiety and critical thinking ability, was not confirmed at either crisis or post-crisis time.

Hypothesis III, predicting a negative relationship between critical thinking and judged duration, was not confirmed at either testing time.

Hypothesis IV, positing the combination of state anxiety and critical thinking to be a better predictor of judged duration than either taken separately, was tested by multiple regression. Results confirmed the significant effect of state anxiety during post-crisis, but not during crisis (Table 2).

Hypotheses predicting significant differences in variable levels between crisis and post-crisis testings wre tested by the t test for correlated means (Table 2).

Hypothesis V, predicting a higher level of state anxiety during crisis than at the post-crisis time, was confirmed.

Hypothesis VI, positing a lower level of critical thinking ability during crisis as compared with post-crisis, was confirmed.

Hypothesis VII, stating that judged duration would be greater during crisis than post-crisis was not confirmed.

Table 1. Correlations Between Major Study Variables During Crisis and Post-crisis

	CRISIS		POST-CRISIS	
VARIABLES	CRITICAL THINKING ABILITY	JUDGED DURATION	CRITICAL THINKING ABILITY	JUDGED DURATION
State Anxiety	.05 n.s.	.01 n.s.	.03 n.s.	.26*
Critical Thinking Ability		.16 n.s.		.06 n.s.

*p<.01
n.s. non-significant (p>.05)

Table 2. Central Tendency, Variation in Scores and Comparison of Means for Major Study Variables During Crisis and Post-crisis

	CRISIS		POST-CRISIS				
VARIABLES	$\bar{X}$	SD (Range)	$\bar{X}$	SD (Range)	t Value	df	2-Tail p
State anxiety	48.7	12 (25 to 33)	33	10 (21 to 73)	11	84	.001*
Critical thinking	60	11 (39 to 84)	64	12 (33 to 90)	−3.6	84	.001*
Judged duration	13	39 (−85 to 190)	5	34 (−93 to 125)	1.7	84	.009 n.s.

*p<.001
n.s. p>.05

Discussion

Overall, variables were found not to be significantly related to one another. There were two notable exceptions, state anxiety and judged duration during the post-crisis testing and state anxiety and critical thinking in the high anxiety crisis group.

The relationship between state anxiety and judged duration was not consistent over the two testing occasions. There was considerable difference in the skew of the anxiety score curve between testing sessions. During hospitalization, the mean state anxiety level for the sample was comparable to norms found for patients admitted to a neuropsychiatric facility diagnosed with acute anxiety reaction; one-third of the sample had anxiety scores one standard deviation higher than norms for the medical-surgical patient population in general (Spielberger, Gorsuch and Lushene, 1970).

The post-crisis state anxiety scores were comparable to each woman's trait score, and the curve was normal ($r = .41$; $p < .01$). At the time, state anxiety and judged duration were found to be significantly related (Table 1).

Orme (1962) suggested that retrospective estimates of time intervals longer than 30 minutes are reflective of a constitutional sense of time, learned over a lifetime and that production measures, or those that request the immediate production of a very short time interval (generally less than one minute, frequently 40 seconds), are more reflective of immediate happenings such as rate of motor or cognitive movement. It may be deduced that judged duration measures a trait characteristic acquired over a lifetime, related to other traits or more moderate level state characteristics. Gorman and Wessman point out that "under different levels of anxiety arousal, different amounts and kinds of cues may be employed in the forming of time judgments" (Gorman and Wessman, 1977, p. 247).

This observation calls for further testing and comparison of time-measurement methods, their intercorrelation and relationship to other state and trait variables. The state characteristic measured by production may be a better indicator of the individual's ability to process the rapidly fed, large amount of complex information normally a part of the hospital-diagnostic experience.

State anxiety and critical thinking, contrary to research previously reported, were not related in this study. However, in the high anxiety subgroup ($n = 25$) tested during the acute crisis period, a significant inverse linear relationship was demonstrated ($r = -.39$; $p < .025$).

Human motivation-performance studies have advanced the idea that a certain amount of anxiety is necessary for optimal performance and for learning to take place. This relationship is curvilinear rather than linear and depicted as an inverted U curve. For the purpose of interpretation of anxiety levels in high stress circumstances such as hospitalization, Janis (1974) hypothesized a curvilinear relationship between anticipatory fear and emotional disturbance after surgery. He found that when patients were categorized according to low, medium, and high fear, the high and low groups exhibited emotional disturbance post-operatively. If subjects in this study are grouped similarly, the moderate anxiety group ($n = 58$) may have been functioning at an optimal critical thinking level. The low anxiety group ($n = 2$) was too small to analyze, but the two subjects did have low CTA scores. The high anxiety group ($n = 25$), demonstrated the correlation between levels of tension and discomfort and cognitive performance. At a certain point on the anxiety scale, critical thinking ability begins to be depressed as a function of high anxiety. Those with high anxiety levels and diminished reasoning ability seem a target high risk clinical group for further study and special nursing consideration.

A positive relationship was hypothesized for critical thinking ability and judged duration. This was not found to be so. It might be concluded that: (1) critical thinking and judged duration are independent of one another; (2) their relationship cannot be described by linear analysis; (3) more baseline measures of cognition, such as memory, need to be examined as correlates of time estimation.

The other assessment method was to determine the shift in the level of variable measures—given the different stress intensities during an acute crisis and six to eight weeks thereafter. With all variables changes occurred in the direction predicted. Anxiety decreased significantly between acute and post-crisis phases and critical thinking improved. Time estimation did not change significantly but did shift in the predicted direction. According to Lavie and Webb (1975), the "indifference interval" or estimate relative to real time (accuracy) lies in the ± 10 percent range. If the sample for the present study is divided according to such a standard, where above 10 percent is considered overestimation and under 10 percent is underestimation, then in the present study, proportional shifts in judged duration given crisis and post-crisis conditions occurred as follows: overestimation was reduced by 12 percent; accuracy of estimate increased by 6 percent and underestimation was increased by 5 percent. Although not significant, the shift occurred as hypothesized and according to theoretical rationale and results of other studies.

Conclusions

The main conclusions drawn from results of this study are that:

• Critical thinking or general reasoning ability was substantially reduced at the time of hospitalization when compared with six to eight weeks post-discharge. Reasoning ability was depressed during a phase when critical decisions were demanded from patients such as those related to informed consent, choice of one to two step surgical procedure, and decisions regarding adjuvant therapy.

• Anxiety levels of patients prior to knowledge of diagnostic results were extremely high. Group average was above norms for acutely ill psychiatric patients and one-third of the group scored one standard deviation or more above the norms for medical-surgical patient populations. Six to eight weeks following biopsy, when the condition was diagnosed benign, state anxiety levels were found significantly reduced and in line with trait anxiety measures taken on both occasions.

• Those women falling into the high anxiety category were found to have positively correlated CTA scores. This means that above a certain anxiety level, patients had increasing difficulty in the reasoning process and in decision-making. Analysis of this substantial group categorized such patients as high risk and in need of special support measures.

• Although judged duration, a measure of information processing capacity, was not found to be significantly changed between the hospital and post-discharge periods, scores did shift in the hypothesized direction. Further, those patients who overestimated time seemed to have the most difficulty absorbing the intense, fast-paced sensory stimulation, a standard of hospital routine. These patients seemed more easily distracted and less able to concentrate than those with more accurate or underestimated judged duration scores. Judged duration may reflect a consitutional or learned sense of time and be considered a trait characteristic related to state anxiety only during non-stressful times.

Those patients with high anxiety, low critical thinking ability, and low capacity for information processing may constitute a high risk group in need of special attention. Those patients with high anxiety and moderate cognitive scores represented another special interest group, as did those with skewed general reasoning ability. It was concluded that each variable seemed related in an important way to the individual's total coping process.

Weisman and Worden (1976) have defined the major concerns of people following cancer diagnosis and determined that effectiveness of coping strategies and good follow-up support are essential to quantitative and qualitative survival. In light of their findings, the conclusions of this study generate a number of research questions.

Since variables were not found to be related but assumed to be important to the total coping process, it is possible that these scores or a combination of scores could be related to coping effectiveness during crisis. Might such combinations be related to major concerns that people have over the course of a crisis? Could a profile classification of critical cognitive and affective variables be predictive of high risk individuals following cancer diagnosis? If so, a profile classification of cancer patients would be a useful tool.

It became apparent that norms for instruments measuring variables critical to the coping process have not been well established. Neither norms for populations in crisis such as cancer patients nor norms where intra-individual comparisons are made over time, stage of life and/or differing conditions are available currently. Would the same results emerge with a male population? Does age constitute a factor? Do one or more of these variables determine choice of coping strategies and their effectiveness?

Four additional studies have been planned to explore these questions. The first is a replication of this study but with a sample of men experiencing diagnosis of genito-urinary carcinoma. The study employs the additional measure of time production and is currently in the data collection phase. The next study has been designed to construct a Stress-Coping Profile Classification (SCPC) predictive of coping quality and major concerns over the first year after initial cancer diagnosis. The fourth study will construct a clinical assessment battery to determine patients' profiles on hospital admission. The fifth study will establish intervention protocols tailored to each profile with special attention to those considered high risk in terms of survival.

Results of this series of studies are anticipated to provide increased understanding of behavior of people experiencing the crisis of cancer and lead to the identification of high risk individuals in need of better, more intense nursing support. **NR**

References

AMERICAN CANCER SOCIETY. *1981 Cancer Facts and Figures.* New York, The Society, 1980.

BADDELEY, A. D. Reduced body temperature and time estimation. *Am J Psychol* 79:465-479, 1966.

BEIER, E. G. The effect of induced anxiety on flexibility of intellectual functioning. *Psychol Monog* 65 (Whole No. 321):1-26, 1951.

BLOOM, V. Definitional aspects of the crisis concept. *J Consult Psychol* 27:498-502, Nov.-Dec. 1963.

DOOB, L. *Patterning of Time.* New Haven, Yale University Press, 1971.

ESON, M. E., AND KAFKA, J. S. Diagnostic implications of a study in time perception. *J Gen Psycol* 46:169-183, Apr. 1952.

GORMAN, B. S., AND WESSMAN, A. E., EDS. *The Personal Experience of Time.* New York, Plenum Press, 1977.

HAMBURGER, M. *A Revised Occupational Scale for Rating Socioeconomic Class.* New York, Teachers College, Columbia University, 1957.

HOAGLAND, H. Some biochemical considerations of time. IN *The Voices of Time,* ed. by J. T. Fraser. New York, Braziller, 1966, pp. 312-329.

_____. The physiological control of judgments of duration: Evidence for a chemical clock. *J Gen Psychol* 9:267-287, Oct. 1933.

JANIS, I. L. *Psychological Stress.* New York, Academic Press, 1974.

LAVIE, P., AND WEBB, W. B. Time estimates in a long-term time-free environment. *Am J Psychol* 88(2):177-186, June 1975.

LAZARUS, R. S. The stress and coping paradigm. IN *The Critical Evaluation of Behavioral Paradigms for Psychiatric Science.* Papers presented at the conference hosted by the University of Washington, Seattle, Nov. 3-6, 1978.

_____, AND AVERILL, J. R. Emotion and cognition: With special reference to anxiety. IN *Anxiety: Current Trends in Theory and Practice. Volume 1,* ed. by C. D. Spielberger. New York, Academic Press, 1972, pp. 241-283.

LEWIS, M. S., AND OTHERS. The course and duration of crisis. *J Consult Clin Psychol* 47(1):128-134, 1979.

MANDLER, G., AND SARASON, S. B. A study of anxiety and learning. *J Abnorm Soc Psychol* 47:166-173, Mar. 1952.

MARTINDALE, C., AND GREENOUGH, J. The differential effect of increased arousal on creative and intellectual performance. *J Genet Psychol* 123:329-335, Dec. 1973.

MAZZEI, J., AND GOULET, L. R. Test anxiety and intelligence in concept formation. *Psychol Rep* 24:842, June 1969.

MEYERS, J., AND MARIN, R. Relationships of state and trait anxiety to concept learning performance. *J Educ Psychol* 66:33-39, 1974.

MOON, W. H., AND LAIR, C. V. Manifest anxiety, induced and digit symbol performance. *Psychol Rep* 26:947-950, June 1970.

O'NEILL, H. F. Effects of stress on state anxiety and performance in computer assisted learning. *J Educ Psychol* 3:473-481, Oct. 1972.

ORME, J. E. Time studies in normal and abnormal personalities. *Acta Psychol* 20:285-303, 1962.

ORNSTEIN, R. *On the Experience of Time.* Baltimore, Penguin Books, 1969.

PFAFF, D. Effects of temperature and time of day on time judgments. *J Exp Psychol* 76:419-422, Mar. 1968.

SARASON, I. G. Experimental approaches to test anxiety: Attention and the uses of information. IN *Anxiety: Current Trends in Theory and Research. Volume 2,* ed. by C. D. Spielberger. New York, Academic Press, 1972, pp. 381-403.

SPIELBERGER, C. D., AND OTHERS. *STAI Manual.* Palo Alto, Calif., Consulting Psychologists Press, 1970.

TENNYSON, R. D., AND BOUTWELL, R. C. Pretask versus within-task anxiety measures in predicting performance on a conceptual acquisition task. *J Educ Psychol* 65:88-92, Aug. 1973.

TENNYSON, R.D., AND WOOLLEY, F. R. Interaction of anxiety with performance on two levels of task difficulty. *J Educ Psychol* 62:463-467, Dec. 1971.

THATCHER, R. W., AND JOHN, E. R. *Foundations of Cognitive Processes, Volume 1.* New York, John Wiley & Sons, 1977.

TOWNSEND, C. M., JR. Breast lumps. *Clin Symposia* 32(2):3-29, 1980.

WATSON, G., AND GLASER, E. M. *Manual for Forms YM and ZM: Watson-Glaser Critical Thinking Appraisal.* New York, Harcourt, Brace and World, 1964.

WEISMAN, A. D., AND WORDEN, J. W. *Coping and Vulnerability in Cancer Patients.* Boston, Project Omega, Department of Psychiatry, Harvard Medical School, 1976.

ARTICLE FOR PRACTICE WITH IDENTIFICATION
OF THEORETICAL FRAMEWORK

O'Brien, M. T. (1993). Multiple sclerosis: The relationship among self-esteem, social support, and coping behavior. *Applied Nursing Research, 6*(2), 54–63.

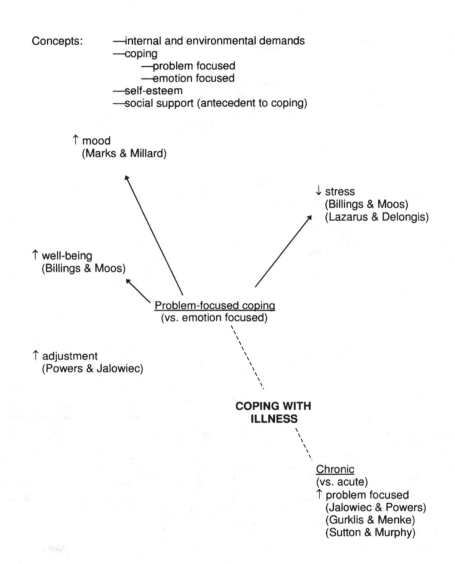

FIGURE B.3   Axiomatic propositions from the cited literature. Model of stress and coping by Lazarus.

Original Articles

Multiple Sclerosis: The Relationship Among Self-Esteem, Social Support, and Coping Behavior

Mary T. O'Brien

This study examines the relationship of self-esteem and social support to problem-focused coping behavior of 101 individuals with multiple sclerosis, a chronic progressive disease. Results included a significant relationship between self-esteem and problem-focused coping; a nonsignificant relationship between social support and problem-focused coping; and that self-esteem and social support taken together did not contribute significantly to problem-focused coping. Although the most frequently used coping strategies employed were problem focused, subjects did use combinations of problem- and emotion-focused strategies to deal with stressful encounters. The findings highlight the importance of assessing self-esteem, social support. and coping behavior of persons afflicted with multiple sclerosis and thus with the ever present potential for physical deterioration.
Copyright © 1993 by W.B. Saunders Company

A STRIKING feature of multiple sclerosis is that it occurs in young adulthood during peak years of education, career development, family life, and when individuals are assuming many social and economic responsibilities. The person with multiple sclerosis is threatened with many potential losses, including physical independence, leisure and social activities, earning power, and role function. This illness experience with periodic remissions and exacerbations presents an uncertainty that engenders lifelong stress.

It has been hypothesized that adjustment to multiple sclerosis is affected by coping behavior (Foley, Bedell, LaRocca, Scheinbert, & Reznikoff, 1987) and more specifically, that problem-focused coping behavior is a positive force in adjustment (Marks & Millard, 1990). Yet there is a dearth of

studies that explore coping behaviors of persons with multiple sclerosis. However, studies addressing coping behaviors of the chronically ill with similar disease trajectories are beginning to emerge.

Coping is behavior directed toward managing internal and environmental demands, or both, that tax or exceed a person's resources (Lazarus & Folkman, 1984). Coping responses serve two functions: (a) they are efforts to deal directly with the source of stress, such as altering a situation (problem-focused); and (b) they are efforts directed at dealing with the emotional reaction (emotion-focused). Although the literature suggests that individuals with chronic disease use both problem-focused and emotion-focused coping behavior to deal with stressors related to illness and disability, research has revealed that problem-focused behavior is more often employed. To explore the relationship among illness, stress, and coping behavior, Jalowiec and Powers (1981) studied the variability of coping behavior in response to stress for two groups of patients: one group with acute illness and a second group with chronic illness. They found that subjects with chronic illness used

From the College of Nursing, University of Massachusetts at Boston, Boston, MA.

Mary T. O'Brien, PhD, RN: Assistant Professor, College of Nursing, University of Massachusetts at Boston.

Address reprint requests to Mary T. O'Brien, PhD, RN, 89 Walnut St, Newton, MA 02160.

Copyright © 1993 by W.B. Saunders Company
0897-1897/93/0602-0002$5.00/0

more problem-focused coping than did the subjects with acute illness. Studies of renal dialysis and renal transplant patients also showed that subjects employed more problem-focused than emotion-focused behavior (Gurklis & Menke, 1988; Sutton & Murphy, 1989).

Additionally, problem-focused coping has been viewed as more efficacious and conducive to well-being (Billings & Moos, 1981; Lazarus & Folkman, 1984) and adjustment (Powers & Jalowiec, 1987). Moreover, in situations of long-term illness, it is associated with less stress and thus implicitly, a healthier form of coping (Billings & Moos, 1981; Lazarus & Delongis, 1983) rather than emotion-focused coping. For example, in their study of adjustment of individuals with multiple sclerosis, Marks and Millard (1990) found that problem-focused coping was significantly correlated with the mood states for composure, confidence, and rationality.

The theory of stress and coping as proposed by Lazarus and Folkman (1984) provided the framework for the integration of the study variables. Lazarus (1966) pointed out that high levels of self-esteem, reflective of self-worth, may reduce vulnerability to threat and thus facilitate healthy or adaptive coping behavior. The theoretical and empirical literature suggested that people who generally feel supported seem to have a greater propensity to initiate behaviors that are action oriented than those without such supports. Lazarus and Folkman (1984) theorized that social support is an antecedent that influences coping behavior. If determinants of problem-focused coping could be enumerated, it would lead to a fuller understanding of the rationale for choice of coping behavior. The suggested link between self-esteem (Lazarus, 1966) and perceived social support (Lazarus & Launier, 1978) and the coping process provided the foundation for the development of the following research questions:

1. What is the relationship between self-esteem and problem-focused coping in individuals with multiple sclerosis?

2. What is the relationship between social support and problem-focused coping in individuals with multiple sclerosis?

3. Are self-esteem and social support, when combined, predictors of problem-focused coping in individuals with multiple sclerosis?

In the current study, problem-focused coping in-cluded cognitive and behavioral efforts employed to deal directly with the source of stress (Lazarus & Folkman, 1984). Self-esteem was defined as that component of the self-concept that reflects an individuals's sense of value, worth, and adequacy as a person (Fitts et al., 1971). Social support consisted of interpersonal transactions that included the expression of a positive affect of one person toward another, the affirmation or endorsement of another person's behaviors, perceptions, or expressed views, and the giving of symbolic or material aid to another (Kahn, 1979).

METHODS

Sample

A convenience sample of 101 individuals with confirmed diagnoses of multiple sclerosis for at least 1 year, and not confined to bed or in an acute exacerbation, was selected from local chapters of the National Multiple Sclerosis Society. The sample included 77 (76.2%) women and 24 (23.8%) men ranging in age from 26 to 73 with a mean age of 46.3. The majority of the sample were white (80.2%, $n = 81$), married (57.4%, $n = 58$), and unemployed (83.2%, $n = 84$). Eighty-four percent ($n = 85$) of the respondents were high-school graduates, and 23.8% ($n = 24$) had completed a baccalaureate. The reported annual family income was low, with nearly 29% ($n = 29$) reporting $10,000 or less. The range was from below $5,000 to over $50,000. The majority of the subjects lived with either spouse and children (33.7%, $n = 34$) or spouse alone (22.8%, $n = 23$); nearly 23% ($n = 23$) lived alone. The average reported length of illness reported was 12 years with a range from 1 to 41 years. All of the respondents reported at least one physical impairment. Ninety percent of the total sample reported the occurrence of at least one physical impairment within the range of "usual" to "always." The three most frequently reported dysfunctions involved walking (97.1%), coordination (90%), and bladder function (80.2%). The frequencies of selected problems observed in the sample population are in Table 1.

Procedure

Subjects were recruited from local chapters of the National Multiple Sclerosis Society. A verbal description as well as a written explanation of the study was given to potential subjects. The volun-

Table 1. Selected Dysfunction of Subjects With Multiple Sclerosis (N = 101)

Dysfunction	Never %	Occasionally %	Usually %	Always %
Vision	27.7	57.4	5.9	8.9
Speech	58.4	37.6	—	4.0
Coordination	9.9	40.6	23.8	25.7
Walking	3.8	14.9	14.9	67.3
Bladder function	19.8	30.7	21.8	27.7
Bowel function	33.7	44.3	11.9	12.9
Transferring	32.7	37.6	13.9	15.8

tary nature of the study, confidentiality of information, and freedom to withdraw at any time were assured. Informed consent was obtained in writing. Subjects were given a packet containing the questionnaires and were requested to return them by mail using a stamped self-addressed envelope provided. Of the 157 packets distributed, 117 were returned. Of these, 101 respondents met the study criteria (Folkman & Lazarus, 1980).

Instruments

Lazarus and Folkman developed the Ways of Coping Checklist (WCC), a 68-item scale that lists a broad range of behavioral and cognitive coping strategies used to measure coping behavior (Lazarus & Folkman, 1984). The WCC contains eight subscales: one problem-focused scale, six emotion-focused scales, and one problem- and emotion-focused scale. The problem-focused subscale includes items that are directed at changing the problem, that is, the source of stress. The emotion-focused subscales include items directed at regulating emotional responses to a problem. Items within the wishful thinking subscale refer to behaviors indicating denial or reality distortion. Items within the detachment subscale refer to behaviors reflecting indifference or resignation. Subjects, using a 4-point Likert type scale ranging from ''1-not at all'' to ''4-used a great deal,'' indicated how often they used a particular strategy. Subjects were instructed to identify stressful events that occurred as consequences of multiple sclerosis and to use each of them as a basis for responding to the scale items.

Construct validity for the WCC was established by Folkman and Lazarus (1980) on a middle-aged community sample (N = 100) through factor analysis that produced eight subscales. Reliability was established by testing for item consistency. Cronbach's alpha ranged from .64 to .88 for the scale items. The overall internal consistency for the present sample was acceptable (Cronbach's alpha coefficient = .78).

The Tennessee Self-Concept Scale (TSCS) consists of 100 self-descriptive statements that portray a picture of the self as it is perceived by the respondents (Fitts et al., 1971). Only the Total P-score of the TSCS was used. The Total P-score consists of eight self-esteem scores: identity, self-satisfaction, behavior, physical self, moral-ethical self, personal self, family self, and social self. For each item, the respondent chooses one of five response options from a 5-point Likert scale labeled from completely false (1) to completely true (5).

Construct validity was documented for a normative sample through comparisons of the Cornell Medical Index questionnaire and the TSCS (Buros, 1972). Correlations ranging from .50 to .70 were obtained from a broad community sample of 626 people. Test-retest reliability based on a sample of 60 college students over a 2-week period resulted in reliability coefficients in the range of .74 to .92 (Fitts, 1971). The internal consistency for the present sample was acceptable with a Cronbach's alpha coefficient of .75.

The Norbeck Social Support Questionnaire (NSSQ), used to measure social support (Norbeck, Lindsey, & Carrieri, 1981), contains three major scales, Functional, Network, and Loss. Only the Total Functional Scale was used in this study. This scale consists of three subscales: (a) affect—the expression of liking, admiration, respect, or love of one person toward another; (b) affirmation—the expression of agreement, acknowledgement, or endorsement of another person's behavior or statement; and (c) aid—the giving of direct aid or assistance to another by providing material resources such as money, information, or time.

The respondent was requested to first identify significant people who provide personal support and then to rate the amount of affect, affirmation, and aid that is received from each individual listed. Each of the three subscales is comprised of two questions that the respondent rates, in respect to network members, on a 5-point Likert-type scale from ''not at all'' to ''a great deal.''

The Total Functional score is obtained by summing the ratings of the three subscales. Norbeck et al. (1981) established test-retest reliability for the subscales on a sample of 67 nursing students. Correlations ranged from .71 to .92. Internal consistency also was established on this nursing student sample that yielded correlations between .72 to .98 for the three functional subscales (Norbeck et al., 1981). In this study, an alpha coefficient of .95 was obtained for the Total Functional Scale.

Relevant demographic- and illness-related data also were gathered. Items included age, sex, race, marital status, education, income, employment, living arrangements, and factors associated with diagnosis and treatment. A checklist consisting of seven functional activities known to be affected in persons with multiple sclerosis was administered. This checklist, constructed from a review of the neurological literature, included vision, speech, coordination, walking, bladder function, bowel function, and transfer ability. On a 4-point scale from never to always, the respondent rated each category according to the frequency of the problems experienced. Items were summed to provide one disability score.

FINDINGS

Means and standard deviations for the three instruments were computed for the total sample. Scores on the problem-focused coping scale ranged between 2 and 30 out of a possible range of 0 to 33, with a mean of 16.50. Total P Scores of the TSCS ranged between 280 and 414 out of a possible range of 150 to 450, with a mean of 346.12. Scores on the NSSQ ranged between 21 and 451 out of a possible range of 0 to 576, with a mean of 156.88. These data are presented in Table 2. Multiple regression analysis, a statistical procedure to examine the simultaneous effects of two or more independent variables on a dependent variable, was used to determine if self-esteem and social support together would be more predictive of variance in problem-focused coping than either

self-esteem or social support taken separately. That is, are the combined effects of self-esteem and social support more likely to explain or predict variability in problem-focused coping than the singular use of either self-steem or social support?

The relationship between self-esteem and problem-focused coping was supported in the findings of this study. The Pearson product-moment correlation coefficient was used to determine whether variation in one variable was related to variation in another variable. The Pearson product-moment correlation coefficient between scores on the Total P Score of the TSCS and scores on the problem-focused scale of the WCC was 0.1820; although low, it was significant at the .03 level of probability. This finding indicates that subjects with higher levels of self-esteem used more problem-focused coping than did subjects with lower levels of self-esteem.

The relationship between social support and problem-focused coping was not supported by study findings. The Pearson product-moment correlation coefficient between scores on the Total Functional Scale of the NSSQ and the problem-focused scale of the WCC was .126, which was not statistically significant. This finding was in a positive direction but not statistically significant. That is, as social support increased, subjects did use more problem-focused coping.

The findings from this study did not support the combination of self-esteem and social support as predictors of problem-focused coping. To test the statistical significance of the contribution made by each independent variable, they were entered into the multiple regression equation simultaneously. The analysis was not significant, $F(2,9) = 2.2048$, $(p = .05)$. The coefficient of multiple determination ($r^2 = .043$), a statistical measure used when 2 or more independent variables (self esteem and social support) are used to predict a dependent variable (problem-focused coping), indicated that 4.3% of the variance in problem focused coping may be explained by the association of self-esteem and social support. That is, the combined influence of self-esteem and social support can account for a proportion of the variance in problem-focused coping. However, the addition of social support accounted for less than 1% of th variance in problem-focused coping. These find ings indicate that the combined effects of self esteem and social support are not predictors o

Table 2. Mean, Median, Standard Deviation, and Range for Self-Esteem, Social Support, and Problem-Focused Coping ($N = 101$)

Variable	M	Median	SD	Range
Self-esteem	346.12	348.00	30.48	280 to 414
Social support	156.88	126.00	88.63	21 to 451
Problem-focused coping	16.50	16.60	6.28	2 to 30

problem-focused coping. Analysis of demographic- and illness-related data showed that problem-focused coping was significantly correlated with education ($r = .21$, $p < .01$), and social support was positively associated with being employed ($r = .20$, $p < .03$) and inversely associated with length of illness ($r = -.18$, $p < .02$). These findings indicate that subjects with more education used more problem-focused coping than did subjects with less education, that those subjects who were employed reported more perceived social support than did subjects who were not employed, and that subjects with longer periods of illness in years perceived less social support than those subjects reporting shorter periods of illness.

To shed further light on the study population, additional analysis was conducted to explore emotion-focused coping behavior. Two emotion-focused scales of the WCC were chosen for this analysis: The wishful thinking (WTS) scale and the detachment scale (DS). Pearson correlation coefficients computed between self-esteem, social support, WTS, and DS showed an inverse relationship between self-esteem and WTS ($r = -.274$, $p < .003$) and between self-esteem and DS ($r = -.172$, $p < .04$). Subjects who reported higher levels of self-esteem also reported using fewer emotion-focused strategies: wishful thinking and detachment. This indicates that as self-esteem increases, the use of wishful thinking and detachment strategies decreases.

The severity of physical dysfunction, as indicated by frequency of occurrence of selected problems, was examined in relation to the major study variables and emotion-focused coping in order to explore any relationships that could provide additional knowledge about the study population.

Results showed a low but significant inverse relationship between social support and physical dysfunction ($r = -.19$, $p < .02$), indicating that individuals reporting the greatest degree of dysfunction had the least amount of perceived social support. A positive relationship between detachment and degree of physical dysfunction ($r = .20$, $p < .02$) was also found, suggesting that with an increase in physical dysfunction, there is an increase in the use of detachment behaviors. Individual coping strategies that subjects reported using were examined. Tables 3 and 4 show the mean scores and standard deviations for each of the problem-focused items and the emotion-focused

items (WTS and DS) on the WCC, respectively. Additionally, the percentage of subjects using the individual strategies is reported. These data showed that subjects used more problem-focused behaviors than emotion-focused behaviors.

DISCUSSION

The finding that self-esteem is significantly related to problem-focused coping lends support to the premise of this study that individuals who believe they are persons of value and worth have confidence in themselves and thus are more likely to employ problem-focused strategies. However, explanation of how self-esteem influences problem-focused coping in persons with multiple sclerosis is needed because of the low correlation found in this investigation.

Because of the complexities of the illness experience with its many uncertainties and its various physical manifestations, situational characteristics may need to be more fully examined, particularly the extent of physical disability. From the perspective of Lazarus' (1991) theory, coping behavior is based on appraisal about what is likely to be effective in a particular situation. For example, if a person cannot change a situation, it may not be helpful to use problem-focused coping, whereas denial or avoidance behaviors may lessen the impact of the threatening situation. Because the self-esteem of persons with multiple sclerosis is probably threatened by chronic physical disease, the relationship between self-esteem and problem-focused coping may vary depending on the level of disability. As shown in Table 1, subjects in this study reported a wide range of functional impairments from minimal to severe levels of dysfunction.

In this study, social support was not a significant predictor of problem-focused coping. There are several plausible explanations. It may be that not all types of social support encourage problem-focused coping. Recently Wineman (1990), who studied the role of social support in adaptation to multiple sclerosis, examined both positive (supportiveness) and negative (unsupportiveness) dimensions of social support. It was found that types of unsupportive interactions (dissatisfaction with social support received) were more strongly related to outcome measures of psychosocial adaptation (depression and purpose in life) than supportive ones. Specifically, perceived unsupportiveness was associated with both an increase in depression and a lower sense of purpose. When the future is assessed as threatening and stressful, and one's needs for social support are perceived as being unmet, stress may be heightened and problem-focused coping may be viewed as futile in light of excessive demands.

Measurement is another factor that must be considered in interpreting findings of this study. Perhaps the NSSQ Functional Scale does not measure aspects of social support germane for a disabled population and consequently failed to differentiate social support as perceived by the subjects in this study. Additionally, a single measurement to assess how people respond in situations that are long-term in nature may not accurately predict coping behavior. Repeated measures of coping behavior would increase the reliability of findings and perhaps tap behaviors associated with long-term chronic disease.

Subjects in this study reporting longer periods of illness and higher levels of functional disability also reported less perceived social support. This finding raises the question of whether social support decreases over time within the context of chronic illness. Norbeck (1981) has commented that support given during periods of crises does not tend to persist into the chronic phase of illness. Situations requiring long-term and continuous support may exhaust the network over time (Norbeck, 1981).

The four most frequently used coping strategies by subjects in this study were problem-focused (Table 3). These behaviors reflect strategies for maintaining control. They suggest that subjects were struggling to solve problems and meet demands that evolved from their illness experience. These findings are consistent with behaviors found in coping studies of hypertensive (Jalowiec & Powers, 1981), renal transplant (Sutton & Murphy, 1989), and hemodialysis (Gurklis & Menke, 1988) patients. From the perspective of stress and coping theory, problem-focused coping is more likely to be used in situations appraised as being amenable to change. The high level of problem-focused behaviors used by subjects in this study suggests that subjects, on the average, perceived their situations as being within their power to manage.

The majority of subjects in this study did use some degree of emotion-focused behavior, and

Table 3. Mean Scores of the Problem-Focused Coping Items on the WCC and Percent of Individuals Who Used the Coping Strategy (N = 101)

Coping Strategy	M	SD	% of U
I try to analyze the problem in order to understand it better.	2.04	.92	94
I try to keep my feelings from interfering with other things too much.	1.80	.95	92
I come up with a couple of different solutions to the problem.	1.49	1.02	90
I know what has to be achieved, so I am doubling my efforts to make things work.	1.67	.96	89
I stand my ground and fight for what I want.	1.62	1.09	84
I go over in my mind what I will say or do.	1.64	1.04	84
I change something so things will turn out all right.	1.53	1.07	82
I try to see things from the other person's point of view.	1.44	1.13	73
I am making a plan of action and following it.	1.26	1.08	71
I try not to act too hastily or follow my first hunch.	1.01	.88	70
I draw on my past experiences; I was in a similar situation before.	.97	1.07	55

therefore it is important not to lose sight of the fa that it played a role in their coping repertoire. Th inverse relationship between emotion-focused cop ing and self-esteem suggests that subjects wi lower self-esteem may lack the self-confidenc necessary to initiate more action-oriented behav iors and thus resorted to employing strategies regulate emotions and minimize disturbing aspec of their situation. Emotion-focused coping al was significantly related to physical disabilit That is, subjects with greater functional disabili were more likely to employ the emotion-focuse strategies of detachment and wishful thinking d rected toward lessening or alleviating emotion distress. Although an explanation is not readi evident, it probably reflects the impact of chron disease on the appraisal of coping options avai able. Because the majority of subjects in this stud

Table 4. Mean Scores the Emotion-Focused Coping Items (Wishful Thinking, Detachment) on the WCC and Percent of Individuals Who Used the Strategy (N = 101)

Coping Strategy	M	SD	% of Use
Wishful Thinking			
I wish that I can change what is happening or how I feel.	1.87	1.01	88
I have fantasies or wishes about how things might be.	1.52	1.11	79
I wish that the situation would go away or somehow be over.	1.72	1.15	76
I daydream or imagine a better time or place than the one where I am.	1.40	1.13	72
I hope a miracle will happen.	1.49	1.25	61
Detachment			
I accept it because nothing can be done.	1.62	1.10	83
I feel that time will make a difference—the only thing to do is to wait.	1.51	1.81	81
I go on as if nothing is happening.	1.23	1.08	69
I try to forget the entire thing.	.95	1.07	62
I go along with fate; sometimes I just have bad luck.	1.10	1.09	62
I am waiting to see what will happen before doing anything.	1.01	1.05	62

reported at least three physical disabilities, they may not have had the energy to cope in an active fashion and thus resorted to more passive forms of coping. According to Lazarus and Folkman (1984), health and energy facilitate coping; further, "a person who is frail, sick, tired, or debilitated has less energy to expend on coping than a healthy robust person" (p. 159).

The most frequently observed emotion-focused behavior, wishing to change what is happening (88%, n = 87) (Table 4), may have indicated that the subjects in this study were striving to alleviate or possibly ignore stressful situations related to their disease experience. The second most frequently used strategy, accepting a situation because nothing can be done (83%, n = 82) may suggest resignation, or contrarily, may be interpreted as being realistic in the face of uncertainty

about an unpredictable chronic disease with the potential of deterioration always present (Table 4). When a situation is appraised as having few possibilities for beneficial change, emotion-focused coping is more apt to be employed. Although the actual situation has not changed, the meaning has changed, and therefore so has the emotional reaction (Lazarus, 1991). Lazarus' (1991) more recent work is focused on expanding the theory of stress and coping to incorporate emotion, which is proposed as a focal point of human experience and adaptation.

Although emotion-focused behaviors may have short-term beneficial effects, Lazarus and Folkman (1984) caution that self-deception and reality distortion are always potential features of emotion-focused coping. Furthermore, these behaviors may lead to denial of what is happening and refusal to acknowledge the implications of the situation. This would have particular significance in a chronic disease context where such behavior may preclude compliance with treatment programs. For the short-term, these behaviors may help a person to maintain hope and optimism in order to cope with an untenable situation that might be overpowering if confronted directly.

Lazarus and Folkman (1984) contend that both forms of coping influence each other throughout a stressful encounter and that both can facilitate and impede each other. Although many researchers consider problem solving to be a salient feature of coping effectiveness and successful adaptation (Billings & Moos, 1981; Lazarus & Launier, 1978), others point out the beneficial effects of using both problem- and emotion-focused strategies to deal with stressful situations. For example, Pollock (1989), who studied chronic disease, asserted that when illness is appraised as harmful, individuals who use both problem- and emotion-focused behaviors have better adaptational outcomes than if they use only problem- or emotion-focused behavior.

IMPLICATIONS

In the last several years, there has been an increased focus on the coping behaviors of persons with chronic disease and disability. This focus emerged primarily from recognition that chronic disease is becoming a greater problem in our society. In fact, chronic illness is reported as the No.

1 health problem in the United States. This is due, in part, to advances in medical science and technology that have prolonged the lives of many chronically ill individuals. Multiple sclerosis is an example of a chronic diseases for which longevity has increased. The importance of multiple sclerosis in health care resulted from (a) the worldwide prevalence rate of 57.9 per 100,000 population; (b) its tendency to occur in the young adult; and (c) its chronicity (Adams & Victor, 1981; Baum & Rothschild, 1981). The consequences of a disease such as multiple sclerosis clearly disrupt personal functioning and daily living that may challenge one's ability to cope.

No systematic research related to coping behaviors of individuals with multiple sclerosis has appeared in the literature. To date, research has focused primarily on the physical impact of the disease, with less attention directed toward the social and psychological implications. Systematic study, therefore, is needed to explore the behavior patterns that individuals use to cope with the many ramifications of chronic disease.

The finding of a positive relationship between self-esteem and problem-focused coping suggests that this study sample viewed themselves as persons of value and had confidence to seek resolutions to their problems. This type of coping behavior is reflective of actions directed at solving a problem as opposed to reducing the tension experienced.

The finding that subjects with lower self-esteem used more emotion-focused coping than those with higher levels of self-esteem raises the question of whether passivity was associated with lower self-esteem in this study population. This needs to be further explored within the context of physical disability.

In view of the positive association between self-esteem and problem-focused coping, nurses need to assess the self-esteem of patients and guide them toward recognition of their self-worth. Nursing has long recognized self-esteem as a key component in health and illness behavior (Meisenhelder, 1985). From a clinical perspective, nurses often observe behaviors reflective of self-esteem and therefore have opportunities to reinforce or enhance a person's self worth by assisting in the discovery of strengths and positive aspects of the self. Self-esteem has been attributed to the reflected appraisals or interactions with significant others (Rosenberg, 1979). With this perspective in mind, nurses may act as facilitators to encourage positive interactions between patients and their significant others. Additionally, nurses can convey feelings of value and worth by their attitudes, behaviors, and interactions with patients, thus providing reassurances of personal value.

The finding that social support was not significantly related to problem-focused coping raises several questions. Although it is assumed by many that social support has positive effects, it has been shown that social networks may include nonsupportive relationships. For example, action by others intended to be supportive may inadvertently reinforce a dependent role and therefore undermine independent coping. Nurses need to be aware of the types of social support provided to patients and need to support and direct social support resources that are conducive to assisting patients in developing strategies appropriate to their needs. The lack of accessibility to social support systems is another possible explanation for a nonsignificant relationship between social support and problem-focused coping. Differences in one's social milieu will have implications for the quality, quantity, and reliability of support available. Therefore, it would be expected that accessibility for a population of disabled people may be quite different than for a nondisabled population. Physical disability may influence the formation and maintenance of social ties because of limited abilities or opportunities to interact with the environment and to therefore restrict strategies reflective of problem-focused coping. Nurses need to explore sources of available support and guide patients and families in obtaining the resources needed for patients to effectively interact with the environment. The combination of self-esteem and social support was not upheld as a predictor in accounting for variance in problem focused coping.

A plausible explanation may be that self-esteem plays a role in respect to how one takes advantage of the availability of support systems. It is conceivable that individuals with physical disabilities may refuse support from others in an attempt to maintain independence and to protect their self esteem. Because the physically disabled need strong support systems and yet need to maintain positive self-esteem, further study is warranted to examine this population in respect to coping, self esteem, and social support.

For persons living with multiple sclerosis who must face an uncertain future, having a supportive network of family and friends provides a sense of belonging and a certain amount of security. Supportive relationships are necessary throughout all phases of the illness trajectory. It is crucial that nurses assess, on an ongoing basis, the nature of social support available to patients to determine needs and types of support required to meet the changing demands of this unpredictable disease. A thorough social support assessment will identify inadequate sources as well as guide the nurse to enhance and mobilize supportive relationships to patients and families who live with chronic disease.

To identify persons at risk for ineffective coping, nurses must be aware of the various coping behaviors used by patients and must be prepared to guide them in more effective strategies when necessary. Furthermore, nurses can best assist patients to cope when they know the patients appraisals of their situation and the coping options available. With this knowledge, both the nurse and patient can set realistic goals to deal more effectively with the myriad demands of living with a chronic illness.

SUMMARY

In this study, self-esteem was found to be positively related to problem-focused coping. However, findings did not support a significant relationship between social support and problem-focused coping, and the combined effect of self-esteem and social support on problem-focused coping was not significant.

Additional analyses indicated some significant relationships between study variables and demographic- and illness-related data. Problem-focused coping was shown to be positively related to education. Subjects with higher education used more problem-focused coping than subjects with less education. Social support was inversely related to length of illness. That is, subjects with longer periods of illness reported less perceived social support than subjects with shorter periods of illness. Subjects who were employed reported more perceived social support than subjects who were not employed. Additionally, emotion-focused coping appears to play a role in the coping repertoire in this study sample. However, generally all significant correlations were low, and thus findings must be interpreted cautiously.

REFERENCES

Adams, R., & Victor, M. (1981). *Principles of neurology* (2d ed.). New York, NY: McGraw-Hill.

Baum, H., & Rothschild, J. (1981). The incidence and prevalence of reported multiple sclerosis. *Annals of Neurology, 10,* 420.

Billings, A., & Moos, R. (1981). The role of coping responses and social resources in attenuating the stress of life events. *Journal of Behavioral Medicine, 4,* 139-157.

Buros, O.K. (Ed.). 1972. *The seventh mental measurements yearbook.* Highland Park, NJ: Gryphon Press.

Fitts, W., Adams, J., Radford, G., Richard, W., Thomas, M., & Thompson, W. (1971). *The self concept and self-actualization.* Nashville, TN: Counselor Recording & Tests.

Foley, F., Bedell, J., LaRocca, N., Scheinbert, L., & Reznikoff, M. (1987). Efficacy of stress-inoculation training in coping with multiple sclerosis. *Journal of Consulting and Clinical Psychology, 55,* 919-922.

Folkman, S., & Lazarus, R.S. (1980). An analysis of coping in a middle-aged community sample. *Journal of Health & Social Behavior, 21,* 219-239.

Gurklis, J.A., & Menke, E.M. (1988). Identification of stressors and use of coping methods in chronic hemodialysis patients. *Nursing Research, 37,* 236-239.

Jalowiec, A., & Powers, M. (1981). Stress and coping in hypertensive and emergency room patients. *Nursing Research, 30,* 10-15.

Kahn, R. (1979). Aging and social support. In M. Riley (Ed.), *Aging from birth to death: Interdisciplinary perspectives* (pp. 77-99). Boulder, CO: Westview Press.

Lazarus, R.S. (1991). *Emotion and adaptation.* New York, NY: Oxford University Press.

Lazarus, R.S. (1966). *Psychological stress and the coping process.* New York, NY: McGraw-Hill.

Lazarus, R.S., & Folkman, S. (1984). *Stress, appraisal, and coping.* New York, NY: Springer.

Lazarus, R.S., & DeLongis, A. (1983). Psychological stress and coping in aging. *American Psychologist, 38,* 245-254.

Lazarus, R.S., & Launier, R. (1978). Stress-related transactions between person and environment. In L. Pervin & M. Lewis (Eds.), *Perspectives in interactional psychology* (pp. 287-327). New York, NY: Plenum.

Marks, S., & Millard, R. (1990). Nursing assessment of positive adjustment for individuals with multiple sclerosis. *Rehabilitation Nursing, 15,* 147-151.

Meisenhelder, J.B. (1985). Self-esteem: A closer look at clinical interventions. *International Journal of Nursing Studies, 22,* 127-135.

Norbeck, J.S. (1981). Social support: A model for clinical research and application. *Advances in Nursing Sciences, 3,* 43-59.

Norbeck, J.S., Lindsey, A., & Carrieri, V. (1981). The development of an instrument to measure social support. *Nursing Research, 30,* 264-269.

Pollock, S. (1989). Adaptive responses to diabetes mellitus. *Western Journal of Nursing Research, 11,* 265-280.

Powers, M., & Jalowiec, A. (1987). Profile of the well-controlled, well-adjusted hypertensive patient. *Nursing Research, 36,* 106-110.

Rosenberg, M. (1979). *Conceiving the self.* New York, NY: Basic Books.

Sutton, T., & Murphy, S. (1989). Stressors and patterns of coping in renal transplant patients. *Nursing Research, 38,* 46-49.

Wineman, N.M. (1990). Adaptation to multiple sclerosis: The role of social support, functional disability, and perceived uncertainty. *Nursing Research, 39,* 284-299.

Appendix C

Guide to Critique of Qualitative Research: With Examples and Practice Study

A. Title

1. Does the researcher indicate the focal topic and offer a metaphorical hint of interpretation?

B. Introduction

1. Is the phenomenon of interest explicitly identified and placed within a context?
2. Is the purpose of the inquiry clearly stated, e.g., discovery, theory building, descriptive base for practice?
3. Is (are) the research question(s) broad?
4. Has the researcher identified the significance of inquiring about this phenomenon, why it is important to study and why it is important to use this method?
5. Is the researcher's context described, e.g., experiences, assumptions, preconceptions, beliefs about the phenomenon?
6. What is the researcher's expertise in conducting this type of inquiry?

C. Literature Review and Theoretical Framework

1. If a literature review is appropriate to the method and prior to data collection, does it demonstrate the complexity of the phenomenon, provide additional justification and credence for the study, and signify how this inquiry will add to existing knowledge?

2. If a theoretical perspective is used for the study, does it conform to the philosophic orientations and naturalistic axioms of qualitative research?

D. Method

1. Is there an overview of the qualitative method chosen, its philosophical underpinnings, and why it is appropriate for this study?
2. Is there a thorough explication of the details—process and procedures—of the study?

E. Sample—Participants

1. Is the sampling procedure delineated? Is it appropriate for this inquiry?
2. Are the participants, the setting, and the rationale for those chosen to be in the study described?
3. Does the researcher discuss the process of gaining entrée to the setting (informal and official) and access to the participants?

F. Data Collection

1. Does the researcher identify the data collection techniques, e.g., interviews, participant observation, review of documents? Are they appropriate for this study?
2. Are the details and procedures of data collection explicated, e.g., how conducted, when, where, with whom, time per data collection sessions, saturation, tape recording, transcriber, and training of data collectors?
3. Are informed consent and protection of human subjects in qualitative inquiry described?
4. Are data records used during the study (transcripts, field notes, journals, logs) identified?
5. Are problems in data collection, ethical issues, and researcher effects on the data discussed?

G. Data Management and Analysis

1. Does the researcher describe the plan for organizing and retrieving data?
2. Does the researcher detail the processes and procedures for data analysis, e.g., coding, categorization, use of matrices, constant comparison, sending memos, using literature? Is a particular method of analysis identified?
3. If a framework were used, is it clear how it informed the analysis?
4. Are the researcher's decision rules used to thematize the data made explicit?
5. Are the researcher's interpretations, hypotheses, conclusions, or theoretical schemata data based, e.g., supported or verified with substantive evidence and examples directly from the data?

6. Is a clear, descriptive, theoretical presentation of the meaning of the phenomenon as discovered by the researcher provided?

H. Discussion, Conclusions, Implications, Recommendations

1. Are the findings compared and contrasted with existing literature and theoretical perspectives?
2. Is there a comprehensive discussion of the results of the inquiry? Do the conclusions reflect the findings?
3. Does the researcher share their applications and/or implications of insight as they influence present practices and understandings?
4. Are the relevance of the inquiry as well as the findings and the importance to the nursing practice and knowledge building identified? Are they appropriate, based on the findings?
5. Are limitations of the study identified?
6. Are recommendations for further study and/or practice and/or education suggested?

I. Quality and Rigor of the Inquiry

1. Does the researcher address measures used to ensure trustworthiness of the inquiry (credibility, transferability, dependability, confirmability, ethics)?
2. Does the work possess verity, integrity, rigor, utility, vitality, and aesthetics? (Mariano, 1995)
3. Does the work have descriptive vividness, methodological congruence, analytic preciseness, theoretical connectedness, and heuristic relevance? (Burns, 1989)
4. Does the work flow smoothly and offer the reader a sensitive, credible understanding of the human experience? Is it "real," "alive," and yet insightful?

EXEMPLAR STUDY 1 WITH CRITIQUE

Wing, D. (1995). Transcending alcoholic denial. *Image: Journal of Nursing Scholarship, 27*(2), 121–126.

A. Title

The focal topic of the study is indicated in the title.

B. Introduction

The phenomenon of interest, transcending alcoholic denial, is clearly identified and placed within a context of alcoholism, the etiology of alcoholic denial, and assessment of denial. The purpose of the inquiry is clearly stated: "to describe the internal processes that alcoholics experience as they transcend denial" (p. 121). The researcher identifies the significance of the inquiry and the importance of using a qualitative method by stating, "Although alcoholism denial is the most common reason that treatment is not received, there is a scarcity of research that comprehensively focuses on the dynamics of alcoholic denial. . . . We know little about the lived experience of denial and the processes involved in moving out of it" (p. 121). The researcher's context is gleaned from the author's 1993 cited publication, which states, "Denial is dangerous to the extent that it can delay recovery and can result in detrimental effects to both the individual and society" (p. 121). The researcher has expertise in this area and cites two studies (three articles) on her prior work, one of which was a field study.

C. Literature Review and Theoretical Framework

The literature review is blended within the introduction and context of the phenomenon. It meets the criteria for demonstrating the complexity of the phenomenon and providing justification for the study. A theoretical framework such as symbolic interactionism was not identified.

D. Method

Wing presents a brief description of grounded theory methodology, its purpose and major underlying assumption: "the researcher seeks to understand the phenomenon under study as experienced, perceived, and valued by the research participants. Personal and social meaning are of paramount importance" (pp. 121–122). Wing then proceeds to explain the procedures of the study.

E. Sample—Participants

The researcher identified the participants in the study. The processes of gaining entrée to the setting were not described. It is unclear whether the 42 participants who participated in the study were the total number of clients in the treatment center; however, the author does state that theoretical or purposive sampling and a convenience sample of treatment center patients were used (in section on "Data Collection"). Brief demographics and frequency of interviews were included. Wing does state that IRB approval from the employing institution and the treatment center was obtained.

F. Data Collection

The author identified 28 days of participant observation in the treatment center and follow-up interviews of discharged patients over a 3-year period. Some of the procedures and processes of data collection were included, e.g., joining in activities while participant observing, frequency of follow-up interviews, development of an interview guide that links questions to initial observations, the actual interview questions, and the use of theoretical sampling to refine interview questions and determine who needs to be interviewed further. The author indicated that she conducted the observations and interviews. Use of a tape recorder, transcriptions, where follow-up interviews were conducted, and length of both the observations and interviews were not described.

Wing identifies the types of recorded notes taken during the inquiry, e.g., observational notes, interpretive notes, procedural notes, and the purpose of each. Although she mentions IRB approval, she does not discuss informed consent of the participants or potential ethical issues in data collection.

G. Data Management and Analysis

The researcher identified use of the method of constant comparison, and substantive coding, code clustering, finding relationships between categories, theoretical coding, and theoretical saturation to analyze the data and develop the emerging theory. She discussed her decision rules for clustering codes to develop categories, and for relating categories.

Wing identified the basic social process theory of transcending alcoholic denial as emerging from this inquiry. The "Findings" section of the manuscript describes five progressive stages of transcending alcoholic denial: (1) reaction to the critical event; (2) role disaffiliation; (3) ambiguous anticipation; (4) peer affiliation; and (5) acceptance (pp 122–123). The author elucidates the properties of each stage as well as the consequences of unresolved stages. The conclusions and evolved theoretical schemata are supported or verified with substantive data directly from the interviews during the patients' stay at the treatment center (participant observation phase) and after discharge (follow-up interview phase).

The theory of transcending alcoholic denial was presented as a process phenomenon. Each of the 5 progressive stages was described conceptually and defined operationally through explication of stage properties. The presentation of findings was clear and supported by data-based examples.

H.   Discussion, Conclusions, Implications, Recommendations

Wing provides minimal comparison of the theoretical schemata with existing literature and other theoretical perspectives, a shortcoming of the article. She identifies one limitation of this and other alcoholism recovery studies, e.g., studying patients who are in treatment. Included in the article are three appropriate recommendations for further investigation. Two recommendations for practice, stage specific interventions, and helping patients plan a relapse prevention program are provided by the investigator. The relevance of the inquiry and findings are summarized as presenting a theory of transcending alcoholic denial that can help nurses understand this elusive concept, confront denial, prevent relapses, thereby assisting nurses and other health professionals to ameliorate some of the personal, family, and social suffering that accompanies alcoholism.

I.   Quality and Rigor of the Inquiry

In the last paragraph of the "Data Analysis" section, the researcher addresses measures to achieve credibility and confirmability. Ethical considerations and the researcher's potential effects on the data were not addressed.

Wing states that "in grounded theory, the researcher seeks to understand the phenomenon under study as experienced, perceived and valued by the research participants" (pp. 121–122). This inquiry meets that criterion.

Considering page limitations imposed on most journal articles, the work as presented appears structurally sound, with a logical research rationale. The theory is useful for practice and makes a contribution to our understanding of denial in the field of alcoholism. However, there is minimal comparison of this theory with extant literature and theory. The researcher demonstrates a knowledge of the grounded theory method and provides a conceptual substantive theoretical schema.

Transcending Alcoholic Denial

Donna Marie Wing

Denial is a characteristic of alcoholism and other drug addictions that must be appreciated in order to understand the recovery process. The purpose of this field study was to describe the internal processes that alcoholics experience as they transcend denial. Grounded theory methods guided data collection and analysis. The author observed and interviewed 42 patients in an inpatient alcoholism treatment facility, then followed 30 participants over a 3-year period. Using the constant comparison method of data analysis, a basic social process theory of transcending alcoholic denial emerged. The theory has five progressive stages: reacting to the critical event; role disaffiliation; ambiguous anticipation; peer affiliation; and acceptance. The theory also elucidates consequences of unresolved stages.

[Keywords: alcoholism; denial]

*   *   *

Alcoholism is a disease that can be treated effectively, though recovery data are discouraging. Approximately 90% of those afflicted with the disease fail to seek any form of help (Nathan, 1988). Although alcoholism denial is the most common reason that treatment is not received (Bartek, Lindeman, Newton, Fitzgerald, & Hawks, 1988), there is a scarcity of research that comprehensively focuses on the dynamics of alcoholic denial.

Within the field of alcoholism, denial is the inability or unwillingness to acknowledge that a problem with alcohol exists and that some form of treatment is needed to deal with it. Denial is dangerous to the extent that it can delay recovery and can result in detrimental effects to both the individual and society (Wing & Hammer-Higgins, 1993). It is a characteristic of alcoholism and other drug addictions that must be appreciated in order to understand the recovery process.

Explanations for the etiology of alcoholic denial have been offered by various disciplines. For example, denial has been viewed as a biological defect (Alterman, 1981; Tarter, Alterman & Edwards, 1984); as a psychological defense mechanism (Anderson, 1981); as a cultural and anthropological phenomenon (Denzin, 1987); and as a sociological interpersonal process (Brissett, 1988). Within the domain of nursing practice, denial is interpreted as a healthy coping mechanism that assists the patient to adapt to a threatening situation (Forchuk & Westwall, 1987). Yet, a sustained state of alcoholic denial prevents the voluntary seeking of treatment and fosters an unhealthy and dangerous state. Denial interferes with the development of effective working relationships between alcoholic patients and nurses.

The effective assessment of denial is considered to be the first and most crucial step of alcoholism treatment (Leiker, 1989; Miller, 1990), though this may be difficult to achieve because of the various aspects of denial and the obscure manner in which it manifests itself. There is the denial of the drinking itself, denial of the consequences of drinking, and denial of the relationship between alcohol consumption and negative outcomes. Because alcoholics have learned to rationalize their drinking behavior, an alcoholic patient may offer a somewhat convincing argument that no alcohol-related problem exists. Some alcoholics may refuse to stop drinking even after becoming aware of serious adverse consequences of their disease (Wing, 1991).

To facilitate the assessment process, some researchers have developed tools for identifying denial (Allan, 1991; Goldsmith & Green, 1988; Ward & Rothaus, 1991). Although the tools are of great assistance in determining the presence of denial, the challenge facing nurses is how to assist the patient to overcome denial and address the alcohol problem. We know little about the lived experience of denial and the processes involved in moving out of it. Therefore, the purpose of this study is to describe the internal processes that alcoholics experience as they transcend denial.

Method

Grounded theory methods guided data collection and analysis in this field study. Grounded theory is a systematic way of collecting, recording, organizing, and analyzing data collected through qualitative means for the purpose of revealing the emerging theory (Glaser, 1978; 1992). In grounded theory the researcher seeks to understand the phenomenon under study as

Donna Marie Wing, RN, CDNS, EdD, *Zeta Delta-At-Large*, is Associate Professor and Coordinator, Masters Program in Nursing Administration, University of Tulsa School of Nursing, Tulsa, Oklahoma. The author gratefully acknowledges Dr. Kathleen Knafl for her comments. Correspondence to University of Tulsa School of Nursing, 600 South College, Tulsa, OK 74104.

Accepted for publication November 3, 1994.

Image: Journal of Nursing Scholarship, 1995; 27(2), 121-126.©1995, Sigma Theta Tau International.

experienced, perceived, and valued by the research participants. Personal and social meaning are of paramount importance.

During the summer of 1990, the author lived in an alcoholism inpatient treatment facility for 28 days to learn the recovery process as experienced by alcoholics. After receiving Institutional Board Approval from both the employing institution and the treatment center, the author joined in the activities of the treatment center patients. Her identity was known to both patients and staff.

During the 28 days of participant-observation, the author identified four stages of recovery, one of which was denial (Wing, 1991). She also observed that denial patients were coerced into treatment by the court, employers, or family members who threatened a negative consequence, such as imprisonment or divorce, if treatment were not received. The author then directed her attention to the basic social problem of ineffective treatment related to denial, identifying "transcending denial" as a core category. To learn more about denial, its role in recovery, and the internal process by which patients transcend denial, she followed discharged patients for 3 years.

Participants

Initially, 42 participants (33 men and 9 women) participated in the treatment center study. Three men and one woman were African-American; the rest were Caucasian. The participants represented a wide variation of occupations and socioeconomic status. Men ranged in age from 18 to 65 years, with a mean age of 35. Women ranged in age from 18 to 66 years, with a mean age of 45.

Thirty participants agreed to follow-up interview. Over the 3-year span, 6 participants were interviewed once; 3 were interviewed twice; 2 were interviewed 3 times; 2 were interviewed 4 times; 2 were interviewed 6 times; 6 were interviewed 7 times; 4 were interviewed 8 times; 2 were interviewed 12 times; 1 was interviewed 14 times; and 2 participants were interviewed 16 times.

Data Collection

Data collection included the data accumulated during the 28 days in the treatment center as well as the data acquired during the following 3 years. Of the 42 treatment center patients, 32 transcended denial while in treatment; 10 were discharged while in denial (Wing, 1991). Five of these patients transcended denial after discharge.

While in the treatment center, the author observed behavior that indicated that a patient was in denial (Wing & Hammer-Higgins, 1993), then observed the day-to-day behavior as the person gradually transcended denial or continued to deny the alcoholism. The author then conducted follow-up interviews of 30 participants after their discharge from the center. Participants were contacted bimonthly during the first 2 years of the study and quarterly during the third year. Most interviews were conducted in person. Five of the participants were interviewed by phone.

An interview guide was developed that linked questions to the initial observations. Because most of the participants had transcended denial while in the treatment center, the author asked retrospective questions such as "How did you overcome denial?", "When did you first realize alcohol was a problem for you?", and "What helped you to recover?" For participants who were still in denial after discharge from the treatment center, the author was able to observe the actual recovery process, and not depend solely on retrospective data. Questions asked included: "What difficulties are you having?" "What is the cause of your problems?" and "Why do you drink?"

Three kinds of notes were recorded. Observational notes reflected what was seen, heard, and experienced; interpretive notes facilitated coding and data analysis; and procedural notes guided the author in pursuing further avenues and in answering specific questions. The latter assisted the author in theoretical sampling. Theoretical, or purposive sampling, is the process of interviewing participants as the research progresses in order to reveal and refine categories and to clarify the emerging theory (Chenitz & Swanson, 1986; Glaser, 1992). Because a convenience sample of treatment center patients was used in this study, theoretical sampling assisted the author in refining interview questions and determining which participants needed to be interviewed further.

Data Analysis

Data collection and analysis occurred simultaneously using the constant comparison method (Glaser, 1978; 1992). First, a line-by-line analysis of the data was conducted to determine substantive codes. For example, "refusal to change," "listening to others," and "altered self-concept" were initial substantive codes. Second, similar codes were clustered together to develop categories. For example, "altered self-concept" and "loneliness" were some codes that formed the category, "role discomfort." Finally, as relationships between categories emerged, theoretical coding was used to conceptualize how the substantive codes related to each other (Glaser, 1978; 1992). "Role discomfort" became "role disaffiliation" as the properties within the category and the relationship with other categories became clear. Theoretical saturation occurred when all data could be explained by the emerging theory (Chenitz & Swanson, 1986; Glaser, 1992).

Credibility and confirmability ensured the rigor of data analysis (Leininger, 1990). Credibility was achieved by sharing the aggregate results with research participants and other recovering alcoholics and by substantiating the theory against material found in the professional literature. Confirmability, or objectivity, was accomplished by corroborating the theory with nurses, physicians, counselors, and long-term recovering alcoholics who could provide alternate explanations for data.

Findings

A basic social process theory of transcending alcoholic denial emerged from this research. A basic social process is a fundamental, patterned process occurring over time and irrespective of the conditional variation of place (Glaser, 1978). The findings indicate that the process of transcending alcoholic denial has five progressive stages. These are: (a) reacting to the

	STAGES	PROPERTIES	CONSEQUENCES OF UNRESOLVED STAGE
I.	Reacting to the Critical Event	Ascribing meaning Altering self-perception Relating event to alcohol use	Denial
II.	Role Disaffiliation	Vacillating Pondering course of action Anticipating doom	Resignation (Relapse)
III.	Ambiguous Anticipation	Hoping Having faith Trusting Anticipating positive Looking forward to Believing Imagining	Unfulfilled Expectation (Relapse)
IV.	Peer Affiliation	Listening to others Relating Opening up Confiding Following Imitating	Sequestration (Relapse)
V.	Acceptance	Assuming personal responsibility Developing accurate perception of reality	

Figure 1: Transcending alcoholic denial.

critical event; (b) role disaffiliation; (c) ambiguous anticipation; (d) peer affiliation; and (e) acceptance. The theory also elucidates consequences of unresolved stages (**Figure 1**). All participants who transcended denial experienced this process. Participants who reached a particular stage, then relapsed, either stayed in denial or started the process over.

Stage I: Reacting to the Critical Event

Regardless of whether they were coerced into treatment or voluntarily admitted, all participants presented for treatment because of a critical life event. Although all who overcame denial spoke of the critical event, there were those who experienced the critical event and were coerced into treatment, yet remained in denial. The author then asked, "What are the properties of the critical event experience that result in a patient's overcoming denial?" The author unearthed the internal process of: (a) ascribing meaning, (b) altering one's self-perception, and (c) relating the event to alcohol use.

Ascribing meaning was related to participants' perceptions of stressful situations. If the critical event held little discernible negative impact, there was little incentive to change one's perception of drinking. Such was the case with a 48 year old man who was facing his sixth divorce. He had internalized a lifestyle where marriage and divorce were frequent occurrences. His being in treatment was a result of his wanting to keep his wife happy, though he had no desire to stop drinking.

Altering one's self-perception occurred when the individual had a firmly identified sense of self that was disrupted by the critical event. This self perception was threatened as a disjunction existed between what the participant was experiencing and the view of self. Some examples were a successful, highly respected entrepreneur who was arrested and faced criminal charges, and a 21-year-old star athlete with a promising future who was dismissed from school because of failing grades.

The third property, relating the critical event to alcohol use, was the turning point that precipitated an early awareness that alcohol might be a problem. When there were no other people or events to blame for the critical event, the individual was left facing the alcohol problem. This occurred to a 36 year old female participant who experienced a car accident and subsequent arrest. These events resulted in an altered self-perception; a homemaker and mother of two was now in prison. Initially, the woman did not see a relationship between the events and her drinking, blaming the accident and arrest on the other driver and an unfair police officer. As witnesses confirmed the police report, and as lab reports confirmed an elevated blood alcohol level, each explanation was eliminated. The woman was then able to associate her drinking with the accident.

All three properties of ascribing meaning, altering one's self-perception, and relating the critical event to alcohol were present for the alcoholic to begin to transcend denial. If these properties were absent, or if only one or two of these properties were present, the patient remained in a sustained state of denial (**Figure 1**).

Stage II: Role Disaffiliation

The participant moved into Stage II, role disaffiliation, when the relationship between the critical event and drinking was perceived. The altered self-perception resulted in feelings of immense fear and confusion as what once was a predictable and familiar lifestyle was transformed into something unknown and erratic. A new identity could not be embraced because the participants did not know what that identity was to be. This stage was characterized by properties of vacillating ("maybe I am an alcoholic, maybe I'm not"), pondering what action to take, and anticipating doom when thinking about the future. The following statement from an 18-year-old male patient exemplifies role disaffiliation.

> Jail was a humbling experience. When you've realized you lost your education, your money, your home, and you spend time with criminals, you realize how bad things have gotten. I dropped out of school. My friends are graduating. I don't have a job or a future. Things don't matter. There's not a whole lot to look forward to. All my dreams are gone. I don't know if it will do me any good to stay sober. I don't want to go back to drinking, but what else can I do?

Two distinct strategies for coping with alcoholism were used by participants in this stage—initiating change and resigning. Initiating change was used by those who were able to tolerate ambiguity. These participants reluctantly worked at changing their behavior, first, by not drinking, then by doing things such as staying away from bars and removing alcohol from their homes.

Participants who lacked a tolerance for ambiguity and faith in their ability to effect change experienced resignation. Resignation was characterized by the knowledge that alcohol was causing great personal hardship and an early awareness of continued negative experiences, but also by an attitude of "that's the way it is." An example of this thinking by a 43-year-old male participant follows:

I have been in and out of treatment centers for many years. I want to quit drinking and I'm honest about quitting, but I just can't give up my old way of living. I had gone a whole week without a drink and was really trying. I got mad at something and the next thing I knew I was in a hotel room with a bottle of whiskey and three prostitutes. They took all my money. These things seem to happen.

Participants who resigned ultimately became convinced that alcohol was not a problem as they continued to experience denial. All returned to active drinking (**Figure 1**). Participants who initiated change remained abstinent, succumbed to ambiguity, and continued to transcend denial

Stage III: Ambiguous Anticipation ("Waiting in the Pumpkin Patch")

The expression "waiting in the pumpkin patch" was used by a participant when describing his perception of Stage III, ambiguous anticipation. Participants who attained this stage anticipated positive experiences, but were not cognizant of what they would be, when they would occur, and how they were to be managed. This stage was characterized by an early acceptance that alcohol might be a problem, hope that life could be better without alcohol, yet a passive rather than active role in recovery. Many of these participants were "waiting to see what will happen."

Things aren't going too good, but I have faith they will be better. I have to believe that life will be fine even if I don't get my wife back. I'm trying to live one day at a time and not worry about tomorrow. I don't know what to do with the painful feelings. I just keep hoping that something will happen and make it better.

Properties of this stage included "hoping," "having faith," "trusting," "anticipating the positive," "looking forward to," "believing," and "imagining." Participants stayed focused on the present, partially because the treatment regimen dictated it, and partially because of the ambiguity of looking to the future.

The range of expectations of this stage extended from anticipating positive, yet unspecified outcomes, to anticipating specifically delineated expectations. For example, hoping that life would be better without alcohol and looking forward to a new life were vague expectations when compared to hoping to get a job and looking forward to a spouse returning. This 38 year old man's experience typifies the reaction to an unfulfilled expectation.

We first say that we will do anything to recover, but then that old thinking comes back and we want recovery on our own terms. When we find that we ain't getting what we want, we start to see recovery as the bad guy and we go back to drinking. That's why I relapsed. I could accept being an alcoholic only on my terms. When I didn't get custody of my children, I took control and started drinking again.

Participants who experienced unfulfilled expectations, such as the man quoted above, could accept being an alcoholic only on their terms. Unfulfilled expectations eventually led to relapse (**Figure 1**).

To the contrary, participants who were able to anticipate the ambiguous said that the process of passing through this stage was gradual. First, they seized the hope that life could be worth living without alcohol, though they were still not completely sure that alcohol was the source of their problems. Second, they started to get restless in their anticipation. They wanted to see results. Third, they came to realize that they needed to initiate action. With this realization, participants began looking to others for help in recovery as they continued to transcend denial.

Stage IV: Peer Affiliation

Affiliating with others was the hallmark of Stage IV. Properties of this stage included listening to others, relating, opening up, confiding, following, and imitating. Participants who did not affiliate were characterized by isolating, distancing, and avoiding.

Those who affiliated started interacting with other recovering alcoholics who were further along in recovery. These role models shared common experiences, viewpoints, and fears with the participants. Peer role models confronted denial and reinforced that alcohol was a problem. Participants said that at this stage they became earnest about recovering and began to accept that they were alcoholics. The following narrative from a 56 year old woman illustrates accepting.

Q: What made the change for you? At what point were you serious about being sober?

A: The people in AA. They didn't give up on me. They kept listening to me and pushing me. Then, gradually I started listening. I received so much love and trust that I started opening up. Now I want to stay sober.

Allowing oneself to be vulnerable determined whether one took the path of affiliating with other recovering alcoholics or remaining isolated. There was great risk in opening up, confiding, and exposing one's weaknesses. Those who could not subject themselves to the risks of vulnerability took the path of sequestration (**Figure 1**). They isolated themselves from others, stopped attending Alcoholics Anonymous (AA) meetings, and distanced themselves from other recovering alcoholics. Eventually, they rekindled friendships with former drinking buddies. One participant stopped calling his AA sponsor and ceased attending aftercare meetings. He asked that the author not contact him anymore. Later it was learned that he had relapsed and died in a car accident.

Whereas the consequence of sequestration was relapse, the consequence of peer affiliation was transcending denial. Participants who established healthy relationships with peer role models approached the final stage, acceptance.

Stage V: Acceptance

At Stage V, acceptance, participants accepted the alcoholic identity, made a decision to become sober, and established recovery goals. This stage was characterized by properties of assuming personal responsibility for the drinking problem and developing an accurate perception of reality. Sobriety was desired as personal goals became more internally focused and less externally driven.

> I admit I first came to treatment because I wanted to make my wife happy. I had planned to stay sober for a short time, then to drink again. I really do want sobriety now.

For the total of 42 participants in this study, 37 achieved this stage at one point, though 14 have since relapsed. Five of the participants have never overcome denial.

Discussion

Recovery studies typically focus on patient attributes and treatment modalities (Akerlind, Hornquist, & Bjurulf, 1988; Gilbert, 1988; Oyabu & Garland, 1987). This study was unique in describing the process of transcending denial. However, as there are patient characteristics that relate to each stage of transcending denial, one cannot overlook the possibility of linking some of these previously studied patient attributes with denial. For example, Liepman and Nirenberg (1989) found that social networks and supportive relationships can influence the alcoholic in seeking help. The questions can then be asked, "How do social networks help the patient transcend Stage IV, peer affiliation?" and "Would some patients be more likely to transcend denial in a particular treatment setting?" In a study of recovering couples, the author also found that attributes were related to recovery and relapse (Wing, 1992). Attribution studies, therefore, should be examined and synthesized with the stages of transcending alcoholic denial to more thoroughly comprehend the recovery process.

A major limitation of alcoholism recovery studies, the present one included, is that they focused on patients who were accessed through either treatment centers or practitioners. With 90% of all alcoholics receiving no treatment, a vast untapped population exists that, if studied, may reveal additional insights about denial. A challenge facing researchers is how to access this nebulous group who are usually unaware that they have a problem with alcohol. Nevertheless, a full understanding of denial requires that we recognize and study those who are not receiving treatment.

The focus of this study has also been on the alcoholic patient. The nurse-patient relationship and the attitudes and abilities of the nurse can have an impact on the patient's response to treatment (Hagemaster, 1991; Sullivan, 1991). For example, the nurse's ability to instill hope in a patient, may assist the patient in overcoming Stage III, ambiguous anticipation. Nurses' attitudes such as acceptance, understanding, and promoting mutual trust may promote the denial transcending process. Further investigation into the impact of therapeutic relationships on overcoming denial is justified.

The treatment of alcoholism can cause much frustration to nurses and other health professionals when the denial process is misunderstood. The results of this study provide a theory of transcending alcoholic denial. Through understanding the stages of overcoming alcoholic denial, nurses and other health professionals can assess where the alcoholic patient is in the recovery process. Stage-specific interventions can be planned that assist the patient work through each stage. For example, if a patient at Stage I is blaming the critical event on external factors, the nurse can develop interventions that confront alternate explanations and focus responsibility onto the patient.

Patients who are at risk for relapse can be helped to plan a relapse prevention program that addresses the phases of resignation, unfulfilled expectation, and sequestration. Nursing interventions would focus on reinforcing patient behaviors that prevent relapse. A patient at Stage IV, for example, would need continuous encouragement and monitoring of relationships with peers so that isolation would be avoided.

This article has presented a theory of transcending alcoholic denial that can help nurses understand this elusive concept. By confronting denial and preventing relapse, nurses and other health professional can help ameliorate some of the personal, family, and social suffering that accompanies the disease of alcoholism.

References

Akerlind, I., Hornquist, J.O., & Bjurulf, P. (1988). Prognosis in alcoholic rehabilitation: The relative significance of social, psychological, and mental factors. **The International Journal of the Addictions, 23,** 1171-1195.

Allan, C.A. (1991). Acknowledging alcohol problems: The use of a visual analogue scale to measure denial. **The Journal of Nervous and Mental Disease, 179,** 620-625.

Alterman, A.I. (1981). A consideration of the values of alcoholics in relation to treatment. In E. Gottheil, A.T. McLellan, & K.A. Druley (Eds.), **Matching patient needs and treatment methods in alcoholism** (203-214). Springfield, IL: Charles C. Thomas.

Anderson, D.J. (1981). **The psychopathology of denial.** Center City, MN: Hazeldon Professional Education Series.

Bartek, J.K., Lindeman, M., Newton, M., Fitzgerald, A.P., & Hawks, J.H. (1988). Nurse-identified problems in the management of alcoholic patients. **Journal of Studies on Alcohol, 49,** 62-70.

Brissett, D. (1988). Denial in alcoholism: A sociological interpretation. **Journal of Drug Issues, 18,** 385-402.

Chenitz, W.C., & Swanson, J.M. (1986). **From practice to grounded theory: Qualitative research in nursing.** Menlo Park, CA: Addison-Wesley.

Denzin, N. (1987). **The alcoholic self.** Newbury Park, CA: Sage.

Forchuk, C., & Westwell, J. (1987). Denial. **Journal of Psychosocial Nursing and Mental Health Services, 25(6)**, 8-13.

Gilbert, F.S. (1988). The effect of type of after-care follow-up on treatment outcome among alcoholics. **Journal of Studies on Alcohol, 49(2)**, 149-159.

Glaser, B.G. (1978). **Theoretical sensitivity**. San Francisco: University of California.

Glaser, B.G. (1992). **Basics of grounded theory analysis**. San Francisco: University of California.

Goldsmith, R.J., & Green, B.L. (1988). A rating scale for alcoholic denial. **The Journal of Nervous and Mental Disease, 176**, 614-620.

Hagemaster, J.N. (1991). Alcohol and other drug abuse. **Journal of the American Association of Occupational Health Nurses, 39(10)**, 456-460.

Leiker, T.L. (1989). The role of the addiction nurse specialist in a general hospital setting. **Nursing Clinics of North America, 24(1)**, 137-149.

Leininger, M. (1990). Ethnomethods: The philosophic and epistemic bases to explicate transcultural nursing knowledge. **Journal of Transcultural Nursing, 1(2)**, 40-51.

Miller, H. (1990). Addiction in a co-worker: Getting past the denial. **American Journal of Nursing, 90(5)**, 73-75.

Nathan, P.E. (1988). Alcohol dependency prevention and early intervention. **Public Health Reports, 103**, 683-689.

Oyabu, N., & Garland, T.N. (1987). An investigation of the impact of social support on the outcome of an alcoholism treatment program. **International Journal of the Addictions, 22(3)**, 221-234.

Sullivan, E.J. (1991). Chemical dependency in the nursing profession. **Journal of the American Association of Occupational Health Nurses, 39**, 474-477.

Tarter, R.E., Alterman, A.I., & Edwards, K.L. (1984). Alcoholic denial: A biopsychological interpretation. **Journal of Studies on Alcohol, 45**, 214-218.

Ward, L.C., & Rothaus, P. (1991). The measurement of denial and rationalization in male alcoholics. **Journal of Clinical Psychology, 47**, 465-468.

Wing, D.M. (1992). A field study of couples recovering from alcoholism. **Issues in Mental Health Nursing, 13(4)**, 333-348.

Wing, D.M. (1991). Goal setting and recovery from alcoholism. **Archives of Psychiatric Nursing, 5**, 178-184.

Wing, D.M., & Hammer-Higgins, P. (1993). Determinants of denial: A study of alcoholics. **Journal of Psychosocial Nursing and Mental Health Services, 31(2)**, 13-17.

A Heideggerian Hermeneutical Analysis of Older Women's Stories of Being Strong

Margaret F. Moloney

As people in our society live longer, affirming the quality of their lived experience becomes more important. The purpose of this study was to ascertain and analyze the meanings of "being strong" as revealed from within the stories of older women. A Heideggerian hermeneutical approach, from a critical feminist perspective, was the methodology used. The sample consisted of 12 women, 7 White and 5 Black, over the age of 65. A team of researchers analyzed the transcripts. Findings consisted of three constitutive patterns: "Surviving," "Finding Strength," and "Gathering the Memories ... Seeing the Patterns."

[Keywords: inner strength; women's issues; storytelling]

*   *   *

Historically, research specifically focused on women has tended to perpetuate the stereotypical view of women as sick and weak. Normal life events such as menopause have been treated as disease states (MacPherson, 1992). Studies of older women have often focused on those in nursing homes, ignoring the 95% of older women who lead active, independent lives (McElmurry & Librizzi, 1986). Research that does emphasize women's health has centered primarily on women's maternal roles, viewing women solely in terms of their reproduction (Duffy, 1985; Dunbar, Patterson, Burton, & Stuckert, 1981; Woods, 1982, 1988). Therefore, it is not surprising that nurses, physicians, and psychologists, among others, have used male-centered models to focus on women's illnesses and "weaknesses," rather than on women's strengths.

To state that women can be strong is a contradiction in terms, given the historical images of women (Cixous, 1980; de Beauvoir, 1974). However, feminists have begun to create alternative definitions of "woman." De Beauvoir (1974) described woman as "becoming," not as a static creature but as one who changes and grows. Kristeva (1980) and Cixous (1980) asserted that a rigid model of a woman is impossible. Hooks (1984) reminded us that when we say woman, we must ask, "Which woman?" Daly (1978, 1987) urged women to celebrate such negative labels as "spinster" and "crone," and use these names to create new strong images of women. Other researchers have begun to uncover the stories of women who have created lives that defy the traditional images of womanhood (Bateson, 1989; Heilbrun, 1988, 1990; Luttrell, 1989; The Personal Narratives

Group, 1989; Robinson, 1985). These stories have the potential to provide other women with positive models of life experience and effectiveness.

A fundamental assumption underlying this study was the belief that all women in our culture possess the potential for inner strength; that this quality of inner strength is developed through living in the world into which they are born; and that inner strength varies from woman to woman depending on her life experiences. The purpose of this study was to discover some of the possible meanings of inner strength in women's lives. The inquiry sought to elicit older women's stories about times in their lives that exemplified meanings of "being strong."

Background

The term "women's inner strength" has been used in at least one study (Rose, 1990) and has its foundations in other work (Belenky, Clinchy, Goldberger, & Tarule, 1986; Gilligan, 1982; Miller, 1986). Miller (1986) stated that women begin to perceive forms of strength based on their life experiences. However, Heilbrun (1988, 1990) concluded that it is difficult for women

Margaret F. Moloney, RNC, ANP, PhD, *Epsilon Alpha,* is a Nurse Practitioner at Southeastern Health Services-Prucare, Decatur, Georgia. Correspondence to 731 Scott Circle, Decatur, GA 30033.
Accepted for publication August 1, 1994.

Image: Journal of Nursing Scholarship, 1995; 27(2), 104-109. ©1995, Sigma Theta Tau International.

to learn how to live rich independent lives if they do not have role models. Recent research focusing on women's lives and experiences may provide women with new models. Five studies of women's lives provide stories of women's inner strength. Rose (1990) analyzed the stories of nine mostly European-American, well-educated, relatively young women. This phenomenologic study focused on these women's perceptions of their inner strength, identifying such qualities as centering, introspecting, and embracing vulnerability. Connors (1986) conducted a fascinating exploration of the lives of six elderly Irish-American women who believed that their stories were not worth telling. *A Woman of the Land* is an ethnographic portrait of an elderly Australian woman (King, 1989) who made her life by relying on herself. The meaning of spiritual well-being in the lives of 13 European-American Appalachian women was explored by Barker (1989). Finally, Bateson (1989) used her life and the lives of four of her women friends to illustrate the ways in which "composing a life" is like using seemingly disconnected threads to create a tapestry.

Method

Heideggerian hermeneutic phenomenology was the research method used to gather and analyze the data. Heidegger (1962) believed that people are all situated in the world and that their understanding of the world comes from their experiences within the world. Heidegger's approach, which is well-suited to an examination of the meaning of women's lives, was used to identify some common patterns of meaning among the experiences of a group of older women.

Participants were sought who were 65 years or older. People who were physically or mentally infirm were excluded from the study (for example, women who were bedridden or who had a health condition that interfered with communication or the ability to reflect thoughtfully). A total of 12 women, 5 African-American and 7 European-American, was recruited and interviewed throughout 1993. Two of the participants were women I knew slightly; the other 10 were referred by friends, colleagues, and other research participants. Nine of the women were widowed and two were never married. One participant had been divorced earlier in her life, was married at the beginning of the study but became widowed during the study. The participants were 65 to 87 years of age. Education ranged from completion of the seventh grade to a doctoral degree, with the majority having completed 12 grades of high school.

Interviews were conducted in person with 11 of the participants. Because the twelfth lived in another state, interviews with her were conducted by telephone. This woman also sent me stories of her life which she had written earlier. I read these stories before we began the first phone interview. Followup interviews were conducted with 9 of the 12 participants.

A letter describing the research project and a copy of the consent form were sent to most of the participants following an initial phone contact, before the first interview. In several cases, there was not sufficient time between the phone contact and first interview to send these papers. In these cases, the project and

consent form were described in detail on the phone and again in person. Most of the interviews took place in participants' homes. Many of the women made coffee; several offered coffee cake or cookies. I took something with me to one or the other of the interviews, usually flowers. During the initial visit, before we began the actual interview, the other woman and I spent some time getting to know each other. I then began the interview by saying, "Tell me a story, a time you'll never forget, about being strong." Some women had notes which they had prepared. Several had talked with their children about which stories to tell me. Often I was shown pictures, high school yearbooks, paintings, or framed awards. The interviews averaged about 1.5 hours, with very few pauses between stories. Each interview was transcribed, reviewed, and analyzed before the second interview took place; the transcript was also sent to the respective participant for her review before the second interview. During the second interview, the participant shared her corrections and editing with me, told new stories, and provided feedback on my initial analysis.

The data were analyzed using the circular hermeneutic process described by Heidegger (1959) and explicated by Diekelmann, Allen, and Tanner (1989). I read each new transcript, first trying to gain a sense of the overall meaning of the stories, and then wrote a short summary of the interview. Following this, I went line-by-line through the transcripts to identify the themes, gradually grouping these into larger themes. As this analysis proceeded, I also conducted first interviews with other women and transcribed those. During this time, I was also engaged in group analysis of the interview data with members of my research team, a group of qualitative nurse researchers whose assistance enhanced credibility, provided consensual validation, and helped in grouping the themes into larger constitutive patterns.

Findings

The constitutive patterns, and the themes that comprised the patterns, emerged for me from the participants' words. The three constitutive patterns that emerged were: "Surviving," "Finding strength," and "Gathering the memories ... Seeing the patterns."

In most of the interviews, participants began by talking about times that were difficult and then went on to describe their perceptions of the origin of their strength to survive the hard times. Finally, they reflected on what telling the story actually meant and reviewed the meanings of their stories in the context of their whole lives.

Surviving

Four major themes reflected the women's stories of survival. These themes were "Living with loss," "Living through hard times," "Being different," and "Putting it behind you."

All the women told stories of having lost people they loved. They also talked about the loss of a home or sometimes the loss of a way of being. In addition, the stories reflected the losses these older women faced as they began to experience the necessity of learning to live with the limitations of aging: loss of bodily function, loss of family and friends, and the possible imminent loss of home.

Often the stories of loss were the first ones told in the interview, and usually involved the loss of a mate or family member. Ophelia told of how she felt when she heard that her mother had died. She said:

> I almost fainted that night. I was standing and he caught me, 'cause I would have hit the porch.... As I said, the first time I'd ever had a death. And it just struck me, that's my mother.

Many of the stories of survival involved living through hard times. All the women had memories of the Great Depression of the 1930s, as well as World War II in the 1940s, and in some cases, World War I. In addition to their all having memories of not having enough, there were frequent stories of coping with a government bureaucracy that made the experience even more difficult.

Jane, who is now 87, was a young adult during the years of the Depression. She talked about what it was like to live through that time. She and her husband had gone to work in Detroit. When all the automobile factories closed, they moved back to the Midwest to be near their families. She said:

> We sold all our furniture in Detroit in order to have money to come back here.... We just got the bare necessities that we had to have, you know, to live in this little place. It was a nice little place, and lo and behold, we couldn't make any payments, so what did the furniture company do but come and took everything out of our house ... except one company left the washing machine because they knew that we had a child, you know ... well, it just happened at that time when [our daughter] died, so they left that ... even took the linoleum off the floor....

The women who were European-American had a difficult time surviving the economic shortages of the Great Depression. Going to college was difficult or impossible for women then because of the lack of resources and because women were frequently not admitted to universities. But for African-American women facing the added oppression of racism, the struggle was even more difficult.

All the women told stories that demonstrated how being female, or being African-American, or, in some cases, being Southern created constraints in their lives that limited their choices or actually created hardships. For the African-American women, the difficulty they faced because they were female was compounded by racial oppression.

Merrell reminisced about her memories of growing up as the stepdaughter of an African-American sharecropper. She remembered:

> They weren't making anything. He worked on this farm so hard, and then in the fall when the harvest time come around, you really hadn't made anything ... because you were sharecropping.... By the time the White man would take out for the expenses for your farm, and then he had to take your part out of that. And that left you hardly with anything. And you just only had a little money to go shopping once a year for clothes, or things like that. And so it were hard.

She went on to say:

> For my father, if he had been a White man, he would have been making more, and maybe I wouldn't have had to drop out of school to help support the family.... Well, now the true part of it ... it's always harder for Black women. It's harder for Blacks.... I had wanted to attend school longer, but I did not, because I had to start work, to help my stepfather.

Woven through the stories of grief, loss, hardship, and oppression were the women's philosophies of survival. All the women talked about putting difficulties behind, looking forward, and moving on. Jane talked about what it was like to move into her own apartment at the age of 70, away from her daughter. Throughout her stories, one could see how she moved forward, having the courage to make changes, and not looking backward: "So I just said, 'Well, this is it, a change, but I think it's going to be for the better.'"

Finding Strength

The women in this study clearly described their inner strength as a quality that developed out of the experiences of their lives. The hard times and losses were times in which they had to be strong, but it was the everyday events of living in the world that strengthened them. Throughout the stories, there were common themes about the process of finding strength: "Being close to others," "Drawing strength from others," "Being at home," and "Feeling good about myself."

A meaningful part of the lives of all these women was their relationships with other people. The women reminisced about relationships with parents, siblings, husbands, and friends. They told stories of raising children, caring for others, and getting along with family members. They also gave examples of others who had helped them to be strong. Frequently these stories were about learning by example from elders. Many of the stories were about mothers and grandmothers. Marjorie told me about her granddaughter, who is caring for her congenitally ill infant:

> I know [my granddaughter] asked her Dad recently, 'Where do I get the strength to go through this?' And he says, 'You've got a grandmother and great-grandmother that you are following.'

Lugene told me about an older woman she knew, whose words helped her when her husband died and she was planning the funeral.

> One thing stuck in my mind, I just love to sit around old people and hear them talk. You get a lot of wisdom from them.... When [Aunt Sue's husband] died, when somebody would come in the door, she would say, 'Oooh....' and she would break down, and then she'd push open that door and she said, 'Li'l Jean, you cry with one eye open and the other shut because you got to watch everything when your husband dies.' That never left me.... But what she was doing, she was keeping her eye on everything.... I remember when we stayed in the country, people would come and that's when they would steal and take things from you....

Many of the women described having found strength through their faith in God. Many grew up in households that were religious, where prayer was a way of life. Endy said, "I came from a very religious family ... and it seems my mother was always on her knees."

People experience the world as a home and the making of a home is a distinctively human way of being (Heidegger, 1971). Although a house may be a home, there are times when one is not at home in her own house, and times when one is most at home with other people. The women talked of being at home with others and of losing their homes when their family and friends were gone.

There were stories of leaving home, of losing one's home, of staying home, and of coming home. Throughout all these stories was woven the desire to create a safe, comfortable place in which to dwell. The theme of creating a home was a thread that ran throughout the narratives. Often the women talked about how their mothers and grandmothers had kept the home together, providing for children and instilling responsibility and values. Many of the women described making homes for their mothers or grandmothers or of having taken others into their homes. Ophelia told a story of "tricking" her mother so as to get her to move into Ophelia's house and Endy remembered her sister buying a larger house to accommodate her dead sister's children.

Throughout the narratives, there were stories that reflected the women's pride in their accomplishments, in their lives outside the home, and in the care they had given to their children and other family members. Edith told stories of what it had been like to be a nurse educator when it was thought that nurses did not need college education. She talked about continuing to fight uphill battles for this and of how she thought the work she did was a part of God's plan.

Others described the pride they felt in their current appearance, their independence, and their ability to take care of themselves. Following Julia's hospitalization, she was moved to a nursing home. She said:

> Then they sent me for 2 weeks to [a nursing home]. And my doctor said, 'Oh, she'll never go back up to [her apartment building].' Both times now, he said that! So when I went to see him, I said, 'I fooled ya, didn't I!' [laughs].... They thought I wasn't gonna be able to do anything when I got back.

Several of the women told stories of how they had had to be the strong one in their families. In this story, Ophelia was telling about what happened after the death of her mother.

> And my baby sister was here but she depended on me. She said, 'Ophelia, what we gonna do about so and so, what we gonna do about so and so?' WE meant ME! What was I gonna do. So I said, 'I'm gonna wait;' I said, 'Now I don't believe in calling the undertaker too quick and I'm gonna wait....'

This constitutive pattern, "Finding strength," is composed of all the strands of everyday life that gave these women strength. The connectedness with others that is embodied in the theme "Being close to others," the strength drawn from other people or from religious faith, the strength found in being at home in the world, and the pride of feeling good about one's self, are all characteristics that enabled these women to find strength in themselves.

Gathering the Memories.... Seeing the Patterns

The process of telling the stories was a pattern in itself. As the women told stories of their lives, they reflected on what it all meant, and frequently made it clear that they were able to see the meaning only now, in looking back. For many of the women, telling these stories enabled them to reflect on their lives but it was also a way of passing on their stories. A number of the women shared transcripts and tapes with their children. One participant edited the transcript to give to her daughter. The themes that emerged included: "Telling my story," "Having regrets," "Living today," "Knowing my strength," and "Looking back over."

Although in many cases, the stories were about experiences that had occurred more than 20 years earlier, the details were clear and complete. The richness of these details reflected what Heidegger called "the nearness of the far," the experience we have of being taken in our memories or imagination to a place which may be far away in time or space. The details of the stories are also part of what makes the narrative a story. They give form and substance to the memory, so that, in the sharing of the story, the listener is also transported.

The narratives were characterized by poetry, colorful detail, and humor. In this story of Eleanor's, she talked about life with her grandparents.

> Grandma dressed us as she probably did her own children. I wore a Ferris waist with buttons sewed all around the waistline. On this were buttoned long knit drawers, a flannel petticoat and an embroidered white petticoat. Our hygiene consisted of a 'hot wash' from a basin of water warmed in a tank on the kitchen stove, set up on a chair. We were ensured privacy for this function and always admonished to 'Wash behind our ears.'

Finally, the storytellers expressed their feelings and thoughts about the meaning of having told the stories. Merrell, who edited her transcript before our second interview, wanted to have a copy for her daughter because, "I never told my daughter, really, about all these things." For Mabel, as well as some of the other women, telling these stories was an emotional outlet.

The storytelling was also a way to examine life. One of the outcomes of this examination for the women was being able to express regret. This regret was an expression of the understanding that life, and the decisions made in life, had not been perfect. In spite of their regrets, the women all expressed a philosophic attitude that, "What's done is done." Mabel said: "There are some things I would do differently if I had to go back over and do it again. But, basically, I didn't do too badly. I've had a long life and a good life."

As the women reflected on their lives, they invariably began to make comparisons between the way things should be, and the way things actually are. Most of the women were eager to convey their perceptions of changes that they thought should be made in society. This critique usually accompanied details about their present lives, including where and how they now live, their relationships with others, and how they stay involved with the rest of the world. Loneliness was often a theme, the result of the losses of aging.

Throughout the narratives, the women talked about being strong, the meaning of strength, whether they actually possessed strength, what it is like not to have strength, and how their own strength developed. Almost all the women clearly stated they were strong. Merrell, in the opening statement of the narrative she prepared beforehand, said it this way: "I want to talk to you about some of the things I have experienced in my life that have made me strong." When I asked Mary, a very traditional woman who was a housewife all her life, if she considered herself a strong woman, she answered: "I think I consider myself strong. If I want to do something, I do it.... Whenever I do something, I know before I do it that I can do it."

Julia and Eleanor both told me initially that they were not strong. However, later, in the midst of telling me a story about how she had had to be strong, Eleanor said, "But I was just normal." I said, "So being strong is normal?" She replied, "Yes. You do what you have to do, and that's all there is to it. There's no way you can back out once you put your shoulder to the wheel."

I asked several of the women if they thought that there was a difference between women's strength and men's strength. Virginia described women's strength as having to do with "the intuitive part of living." Marjorie concurred.

It's a different type of strength. More a silent strength. Not a macho one. Men's is usually more on the macho side ... although there are some amazing men in their strength, what they do.... Men usually broadcast it a little bit more.

Toward the end of the interviews, most of the women engaged in a summing-up and took a clear look at the present. Several of the women expressed their feelings about dying or about losing their independence. There was usually an expression of having come to peace, of accepting the way things had been in the past and feeling comfortable about the future. Virginia expressed her impressions of her life as a whole, saying, "The high moments and the low moments blend together into a fabric of your life...."

For most of the women, there was a sense that events in their lives had been ordered for a reason, even if it was a reason they could not understand. Edith concluded.

But when you look back on it and you see what happened, and you know what you accomplished wasn't your doings, it had to be in the patterns of things to happen and to come.... When you look back on it ... you see the pattern was there all the time....

Discussion

To understand strength from a woman's perspective can change the ways nurses view themselves and their female clients. Understanding the possibility that an older woman perceives herself as strong, instead of assuming that she sees herself as weak, changes the ways in which nurses assist others. Helping women verbalize their strength may help them visualize themselves as strong in a way that potentiates health.

The stories in this study illustrate the empowering nature of narrative (Diekelmann, 1991; Hartman, 1991; Heilbrun, 1988; Hutchinson, 1994; Sandelowski, 1991). There was often a catharsis at having told the stories. In telling their stories, many of which had not been voiced before, the women also found a way to reflect on the meaning of their lives. There was a sense, through the storytelling, of coming to peace with one's life, as well as a recognition that the wisdom one possessed could be of value to others. Storytelling can be thought of as a way of caring: caring for the individual who is telling the story by providing her with a vehicle for looking over her life, and caring for the listener who gains from the wisdom of the storyteller's experiences. For a nurse to encourage the telling of life stories can be as enriching for herself as for the storyteller.

In addition, for nurses as women to voice their own strengths, and their pride in their work, is an empowering act. For nurses, it can also be empowering to realize that their own stories can give other women "plots" on which to build their life stories (Bateson, 1989; Hartman, 1991; Heilbrun, 1988, 1990).

For the nurse who cares for women of a different race, class, or age than her own, the understanding of how their experiences compare to hers can enable her to help women find and use their strength. Understanding the connections and contrasts of life experiences can also begin to create a better appreciation of others' experience (Lugones & Spelman, 1990). As the number of aged persons in our society increases, seeing beyond stereotypes of the aged and appreciating and honoring the strengths of older women and men are crucial to helping older people.

This study illustrates the value of exploring "life in the margins" (Bateson, 1989; Daly, 1992). The lives of older women are not usually considered worthy of attention; most older women are not important or powerful. The power of these stories and the insights of these women have important implications for the lives of others.

Nurses might also be considered to be in the margins, since most are women and their work is often directed by others. For example, the work of advanced practice nurses is especially marginal, close to the boundaries of mainstream nursing practice and infringing on the boundaries of medical practice. According to Bateson (1989), it is in these margins "where new visions may be born." It is in these margins that nursing research must continue to explore new visions of practice and new visions of health care.

Research methods such as the one used in this study, Heideggerian hermeneutics, encourage the voicing of women's experiences and emphasize understanding the meaning of experience from the individual's perspective. Narrative, in this study, can be seen as a powerful mode for communicating strength, as well as for sharing strength. The use of narrative, as well as the use of poetry and other creative art forms, may have potential for demonstrating women's strengths and the importance of women's experiences. The power of these stories and the insights of these women suggest that the creativeness that lurks close to the boundaries of society has important implications for the lives of everyone. Researchers must save these stories, because as Edith said, "When an old person dies, it's like a library burning down."

References

Barker, E. (1989). **Being whole: Spiritual well-being in Appalachian women, a phenomenological study.** Unpublished doctoral dissertation, University of Texas, Austin.

Bateson, M.C. (1989). *Composing a life.* New York: Plume.

Belenky, M., Clinchy, B., Goldberger, N., & Tarule, J. (1986). **Women's ways of knowing.** New York: Basic Books.

Cixous, H. (1980). Sorties. In E. Marks & I. de Courtivron (Eds.), **New French feminisms** (90-98). New York: Schocken Books.

Connors, D. (1986). **I've always had everything I've wanted—but I never wanted very much: An experiential analysis of Irish-American working class women in their nineties.** Unpublished doctoral dissertation, Brandeis University.

Daly, M. (1978). **Gyn/ecology.** Boston: Beacon Press.

Daly, M. (1987). **Websters' first new intergalactic wickedary of the English language.** Boston: Beacon Press.

Daly, M. (1992). **Outercourse.** San Francisco: Harper Collins.

de Beauvoir, S. (1974). **The second sex.** New York: Vintage Books.

Diekelmann, N. (1991). The emancipatory power of the narrative. In **Curriculum revolution: Community building and activism** (41-62). New York: The National League for Nursing.

Diekelmann, N., Allen, D., & Tanner, C. (1989). **The NLN criteria for appraisal of baccalaureate programs: A critical hermeneutic analysis.** New York: National League for Nursing.

Duffy, M. (1985). A critique of research: A feminist perspective. **Health Care for Women International, 6,** 341-352.

Dunbar, S., Patterson, E., Burton, C., & Stuckert, G. (1981). Women's health and nursing research. **Advances in Nursing Science, 2(2),** 1-10.

Gilligan, C. (1982). **In a different voice.** Cambridge: Harvard University Press.

Hartman, E. (1991). Telling stories: The construction of women's agency. In E. Hartman & E. Messer-Davidow (Eds.), **Engendering knowledge** (11-34). Knoxville: The University of Tennessee Press.

Heidegger, M. (1959). **An introduction to metaphysics** (R. Manheim, Trans.). New Haven: Yale University Press.

Heidegger, M. (1962). **Being and time.** New York: Harper & Row. (original work published 1927)

Heidegger, M. (1971). **Poetry, language, thought** (A. Hofstadter, Trans.). New York: Harper & Row.

Heilbrun, C. (1988). **Writing a woman's life.** New York: Ballantine Books.

Heilbrun, C. (1990). **Hamlet's mother and other women.** New York: Ballantine Books.

Hooks, B. (1984). **Feminist theory: From margin to center.** Boston: South End Press.

Hutchinson, S.A. (1994) Benefits of participating in research interviews. **Image: Journal of Nursing Scholarship, 26,** 161-164.

King, P. (1989). A woman of the land. **Image: Journal of Nursing Scholarship, 21,** 19-22.

Kristeva, J. (1980). Woman can never be defined. In E. Marks & I. de Courtivron (Eds.), **New French feminisms** (137-141). New York: Schocken Books.

Lugones, M.C., & Spelman, E.V. (1990) Have we got a theory for you! Feminist theory, cultural imperialism and the demand for "the women's voice". In A. Al-Hibri (Ed.), **Hypatia reborn** (18-33). Bloomington, IN: Indiana University Press.

Luttrell, W. (1989). Working-class women's ways of knowing: Effects of gender, race, and class. **Sociology of Education, 62,** 33-46.

MacPherson, K.I. (1992). Cardiovascular disease in women and noncontraceptive use of hormones: A feminist analysis. **Advances in Nursing Science, 14(4),** 34-49.

McElmurry, B., & Librizzi, S. (1986). The health of older women. **Nursing Clinics of North America, 21(1),** 161-171.

Miller, J. (1986). **Toward a new psychology of women** (2nd ed.). Boston: Beacon Press. (original work published 1976)

The Personal Narratives Group. (Eds.) (1989). **Interpreting women's lives.** Bloomington, IN: Indiana University Press.

Robinson, C. (1985). Black women: A tradition of self-reliant strength. In J. Robbins & R. Siegel (Eds.), **Women changing therapy** (135-144). New York: Harrington Park Press.

Rose, J. (1990). Psychologic health of women: A phenomenologic study of women's inner strength. **Advances in Nursing Science, 12(2),** 56-70.

Sandelowski, M. (1991). Telling stories: Narrative approaches in qualitative research. **Image: Journal of Nursing Scholarship, 23,** 161-166.

Woods, N. (1982). Women's health: Perspectives for nursing research. **Nursing Clinics of North America, 17(1),** 113-119.

Woods, N. (1988). Women's health. **Annual Review of Nursing Research, 6,** 209-236.

Appendix D

Guide to Critique
of Philosophical Research

1. Is the topic to be explored, its breadth and scope, explicitly identified in the title of the dissertation? Or early in the introduction?
2. Are the purposes and aims of the inquiry clearly stated early in the introduction as well as in the methodology to be used?
3. Is the rationale justifying the inquiry convincing and regarded as worthwhile? Necessary? Useful? And not a duplication without new insights?
4. Does the organization of the inquiry build logically from one topic to the next?
5. Does the inquiry proceed through argumentation by interpretation rather than argumentation by empirical evidence as the major mode of discussion?
6. Is bibliographical data including the author's biases and perspective given if they are likely to influence the interpretation of the major themes developed in the argumentation? Is it necessary for this inquiry?
7. Are all major writings on the question or topic, pro and con, consulted in the presentation of possible views and/or approaches to its resolution? If not, is a rationale given for selection of certain authors over others?
8. Is there a consistency in the use of rhetoric and preservation of the selected author's views in context throughout the dissertation?
9. Are the strengths and weaknesses of opposing positions explicit in their exposition in the argumentation and resolution of the question?
10. Are assumptions and/or presuppositions identified that underlie the major arguments or positions from which they were derived?
11. Do the arguments developed in the inquiry adhere to the assumptions of the positions from which they were derived?
12. Is it clear whom the intended readers are to be addressed in the inquiry?
13. Is the proposal or answer derived through argumentation by interpretation convincing? And intelligible to the intended readers?
14. Are the aims and purposes of the dissertation accomplished?

Appendix E

Issues of Control and Validity: Quantitative Studies

CONTROL OF EXTRANEOUS VARIABLES BY DESIGN—AN EXAMPLE

An uncontrolled variable that greatly influences the results of a study is called an extraneous variable. Extraneous variables are those that lie outside the interest, or perhaps the control, of the researcher. There are usually a great number of these variables present, and they can often play an important role in affecting research results.

Ex. Lindeman, C., & Aernam, B. (1977). Nursing intervention with the presurgical patient: The effects of structured and unstructured preoperative teaching. In F. Downs & M. Newman (Eds.), *A source book of nursing research* (2nd ed., pp. 45–63). Philadelphia: F. A. Davis.

    A. Independent variables

        1. Methods of teaching (symbolized by X_1 and X_2)

    B. Dependent variables (symbolized by O_1, O_2, O_3, and O_4, or observations)

        1. Length of hospital stay
        2. Need for analgesics
        3. Ventilatory function

    B. Controls of extraneous variables

        1. Controlled for contamination by pretest posttest design, contamination meaning that if nurses instructed in structured preoperative teaching

TABLE E.1 Control of Extraneous Variables

S^*, O_1, X_1, & O_2.	S^*, O_3, X_2, & O_4.
Control group admitted 5/24–6/18. Unstructured preoperative teaching. Pretest of ventilatory function. Posttest of ventilatory function, length of hospital stay, number of analgesics, during first 72 postop hours.	Experimental group admitted 11/1–11/27. Structured preoperative teaching. (exercise, breathing, coughing + sound-on-slide program). Pretest (same) Posttest (same)

$^*S$ denotes accrual of sample.

were administering the teaching during the same period that nurses were administering unstructured intuitive teaching, it is highly probable there would be contamination between nurses and between patients.

2. Criteria for subjects

— age was 15+ years
— subjects were admitted under nonemergency conditions

3. Because the site of an incision affects postoperative ventilatory function, the subjects were classified:

— major chest and neck surgery
— minor chest surgery
— lower abdominal surgery
— upper abdominal
— other

The researchers tested for significant differences in frequencies between groups by use of chi square. The groups were found not to be significantly different.

4. Standardization of structured preoperative teaching regimen

— definition of effective postoperative stir-up regime
— formulation of teaching plan that delineated content and process of preoperative teaching
— development of teaching aids for staff development and patient teaching

— retraining of nursing personnel on the surgical units
— consistency among departments of physical therapy, respiratory therapy, surgery, and anesthesia on first two

5. In the data analyses, 3 subjects from the control group and 19 from the experimental group were dropped due to death, return to surgery for a second procedure, or prolonged hospitalization due to medical problems not related to their surgery.

C. Extraneous variables not controlled

1. No random assignment
2. No control of season
3. The actual age range was not cited, only the mean for each group. The age range appears broad.
4. Ventilatory function was evaluated before teaching, after surgery, but not following the teaching
5. Respiratory and circulatory status were not evaluated preoperatively
6. Evaluation of learning prior to and after teaching was not done
7. Ability of patient to comprehend instructions was not assessed
8. Variations between nurses were not considered
9. Postoperative testing was done 24 hours after the time listed on the surgical report for the start of surgery rather than 24 hours following discharge from the recovery room
10. Physicians' orders for analgesics did not allow this variable to vary
11. The type and length of surgery were broad

Appendix F

Testing Hypotheses with an Exemplar Study: Statistical Significance, Error, Directionality, and Power

From: Waltz, C., & Bausell, R. B. (1981). *Nursing research: Design, statistics and computer analysis* (pp. 19–29). Philadelphia: F. A. Davis. Reprinted with permission from the publisher.

Ex. "Consider two groups of subjects, one having received preoperative instruction regarding what they could expect from their surgical experience, the other having received only the usual hospital routine." (p. 19)

"If these groups were to be compared with respect to the amount of postoperative medication they required, then all that would seemingly be necessary to test the null hypothesis would be to count up the number of times patients in each group requested medication and see if one group requested more than the other. Theoretically, it would seem that if the group that received the preoperative instruction requested exactly the same amount of medication as the group that did not receive instruction, there would be no relationship between preoperative instruction and medication requests." (pp. 19–20)

"Under such conditions, the null hypothesis would be considered to be probably true (that is, H_o = 'Patients receiving preoperative instruction do not differ from patients not receiving preoperative instruction with respect to the amount of medication requested following surgery').

"With this particular outcome, such a conclusion would be difficult to refute. What, however, if the experimental group (that is, those subjects receiving preoperative instruction) had requested medication a total of 78 times and the control group's

123

requests had totaled 79? Would the researcher be justified in arguing that the null hypothesis was probably false and that a relationship did indeed exist between the variables? Would a hospital administrator be justified in authorizing preoperative instruction for all patients on the basis of this minute difference between groups?"

"The probability is that after a little thought a reasonable administrator would conclude that the difference was too small to be sure that preoperative instruction had any real effect upon requests for medication. Such a decision would be correct because, in research dealing with different groups of people under different conditions, results are almost never identical across groups, people, and time. Given two or more groups, in fact, it is far more likely that in the final analysis these groups will differ to some degree than it is that they will not differ at all. Given this state of affairs, therefore, it should be obvious that some objective criterion should be available to ascertain whether or not a hypothesized relationship should be accepted as 'real' or rejected as not real. Such a criterion does exist. It is called statistical significance and it is basic to all hypothesis testing." (p. 20)

I. CONCEPT OF STATISTICAL SIGNIFICANCE

    A.   "The substitution of a statistical value for an observed relationship or difference"

    B.   "The comparison of the statistical value to a distribution of other statistical values to determine how likely such a value (and hence the relationship it represents) would be to occur by chance alone

        1.   "If the odds are on the side of the observed relationship not occurring by chance alone, then the H_0 is considered probably false (and H_1 probably true)."

        2.   "If the odds seem to favor the relationship occurring by chance, then the H_0 is accepted as probably true." (p. 20)

    Ex. "Suppose the results in the following table had occurred when conducting the above mentioned study contrasting a group of patients receiving preoperative instruction with a group receiving no instruction with respect to requests for medication following surgery." (p. 20)

"Patients receiving preoperative instruction appeared to request pain medications less frequently than control patients: the former registering 11 requests as opposed to 25 for the latter. The question becomes, since it is unlikely that the two groups would have registered identical medication requests regardless of the experimental treatment (instruction), is the difference actually observed (that is, $25 - 11 = 14$) likely to have occurred by chance alone? If the answer is no, then the researcher can conclude that the observed difference (14) was due to the fact that one group received preoperative instruction and the other did not (if the study was conducted carefully) and that H_0 could be rejected as probably false. If the answer is yes, then

TABLE F.1 Hypothetical Postoperative Medication Requests of Patients Who Received and Patients Who Did Not Receive Preoperative Instruction (p. 21)

E (instruction)		C (no instruction)	
Patient	Number of requests	Patient	Number of requests
#1	3	#5	4
#2	2	#6	6
#3	1	#7	8
#4	5	#8	7
Total	11	Total	25

the researcher would conclude that the instruction had no measurable effect and that H_0 was probably correct." (pp. 20–21)

"The actual decision of whether or not H_0 should be considered probably true or probably false is easy to make. Conceptually, the process consists of two steps: (1) determining the level of error that can be tolerated in reaching the decision, and (2) determining how likely the actual results obtained were to have occurred by chance alone." (p. 21)

II.   LEVEL OF ERROR

A.   In behavioral research, the maximum tolerable error for considering the H_0 probably false is 5% (researchers are willing to be wrong 5 times out of 100 when rejecting the H_0)

  1.   called the "alpha level" or "level of significance"

Probability of obtained results occurring by chance

A.   "Determine how likely the actual results obtained were to have occurred by chance alone

  1.   choose an appropriate statistic to represent the relationship
  2.   compute the statistic (= translating the relationship in such a way that it can be represented by the numerical value of the statistic)
  3.   compare the statistic to its particular distribution to see how likely it (and hence the relationship it represents) was to occur by chance alone."

Ex.   "Given the eight medication requests observed in the study (e.g., 3, 2, 1,

5, 4, 6, 8, and 7), what is the probability that a difference as large as 14 (25 − 11) would occur by chance alone?" (p. 22)

"The total number of combinations of two groups of four numbers each can easily be calculated mathematically (by computer for large amounts of data). Starting with the eight numbers listed in the previous table, it is possible to construct 70 different combinations, of which having the numbers 3, 2, 1, and 5 in the experimental group and 4, 6, 8, and 7 in the control is only one (a few of these combinations are in the table below)."

"The researcher could then compute differences between these 70 unique combinations of four numbers and construct a frequency distribution of the differences between the two groups (see table below). Note that although there are 70 different combinations of four numbers possible, there are not 70 unique differences between groups." (p. 23)

"This frequency distribution represents all the possible chance differences that could occur between the two groups of four numbers and the possible ways in which each difference can occur. Once constructed, all the researcher need do to determine how likely the observed difference of 14 was to occur by chance alone is to determine how many ways a difference of 14 or greater could occur and divide that figure by the total number of unique combinations of two groups of four numbers each.

"Referring to the distribution, it is found that there are two ways by which the difference of 14 could have occurred by chance and two ways by which an even greater difference (16) could have occurred. This means that a difference as great as 14 could have occurred by chance a total of 4 times out of 70, thus the probability that the observed 14 did occur by chance alone is 4 divided by 70 or 0.057. If the level of significance or alpha level of this study had been set at 0.05, which is likely, then the null hypothesis could not be rejected because the researcher would be wrong 5.7 out of 100 times rather than the permissible 5 out of 100." (p. 24)

III. DIRECTIONALITY

TABLE F.2   Examples of Possible Combinations for the Two Groups of Four Numbers

(1)		(2)		(3)		(4)		(5)		(6)	
E	C	E	C	E	C	E	C	E	C	E	C
1	5	1	4	1	2	1	2	2	1	5	1
2	6	2	6	3	4	3	4	3	4	6	2
3	7	3	7	6	5	6	5	6	5	7	3
4	8	5	8	7	8	8	7	7	8	8	4
10	26	11	25	17	19	18	18	18	18	26	10
	16		14		2		0		0		16

**TABLE F.3 Frequency Distribution of Differences
Between the Two Groups (p. 24)**

Differences between E and C totals	Total number of unique combinations that can produce these differences
16	2
14	2
12	4
10	6
8	10
6	10
4	14
2	14
0	8
	70

"In the above study, the researcher tested the following H_1: 'Patients receiving preoperative instruction differ significantly from patients not receiving preoperative instruction with respect to number of postoperative medication requests.' Given this non-directional hypothesis, a difference of 14 favoring the control group would receive the same treatment as the observed difference of 14 favoring the experimental group. A very different situation would exist, however, if the researcher had posited a direction to the relationship." (pp. 24–25)

Ex. "Suppose the following H_0 had been tested: 'Patients receiving preoperative instruction register significantly fewer postoperative medication requests than patients not receiving preoperative instruction.' " (p. 25)

"In this situation, unlike the previous one, a difference of 14 favoring the control group would not receive the same treatment as the observed difference of 14 favoring the experimental group. The reason for this should be clear. H_1 posited a significant (that is, an alpha of 0.05 or less) difference between the groups *favoring* the experimental group, hence any difference favoring the control group would be considered supportive of H_0, not H_1. In other words, no matter how great a difference observed in favor of the control group, H_1 would be automatically rejected as probably false."

"Given the directional H_1 positing a difference favoring the experimental group therefore, a question arises concerning how to redefine differences occurring by chance and consequently how to determine the probability of a difference as large as 14 *favoring the experimental* group occurring by chance."

"The above table can no longer be used because no distinctions were made between the direction of the difference between the experimental and control groups.

Referring to that distribution indicates, for example, that from the total 70 unique combinations of groups of four numbers, two could be expected to produce differences as large as 16 and two produce differences as large as 14. In actuality, only one combination was capable of producing a difference of 16 favoring the experimental group (that is, E = 1, 2, 3, and 4; C = 5, 6, 7, and 8), the other difference of 16 favored the control group (that is, E = 5, 6, 7, and 8; C = 1, 2, 3, and 4) as indicated in the third table above. The same held for differences of 14; only one unique combination of the 70 possible favored the experimental group, the other consisted of a mirror image favoring the control group.

"To ascertain the probability of a 14 favoring E when such a direction had been hypothesized a priori, therefore, the researcher would count only the single difference of 16 and the single difference of 14 favoring the experimental group, and would ignore the 16 and 14 differences favoring the control group. Thus, instead of dividing 4 (two differences of 16 and two of 14) by 70, the researcher would divide 2 by 70 and obtain 0.0285 instead of 0.057, thereby rejecting H_0 as probably false and accepting H_1 as probably true.

"In other words, if everything else is equal, the same difference is half as likely to occur by chance in a directional hypothesis as in a nondirectional one *if that difference occurs in the proper direction*." (p. 25)

Summary:

1. The number of requests for each member of the E group and for each member of the C group are determined.
2. All possible combinations of numbers of requests by E subjects with numbers of requests by C subjects are computed.
3. The number of requests for the E group and for the C group are totaled for each combination.
4. The difference is calculated for each combination.
5. A frequency distribution of the differences represents all the possible chance differences that could occur and the possible ways in which each difference can occur.

   Assumption: In a nondirectional hypothesis, the direction is not considered. E = 10; C = 14; difference = −4. (Those who have preop teaching will make fewer requests.) Also included, however, is E = 14; C = 10; difference = +4.

6. The researcher now can determine how likely the observed difference between the E group and C group in *their* study could occur by chance alone.

   Procedure: Divide the calculated difference by the total number of unique combinations. If the value is less than the set alpha, or significance level, H_0 can be rejected. (The researcher has been wrong less than 5 times out of 100 if *p* is set at .05 and the above value is less.)

7. In the case of a directional hypothesis, a difference favoring the C group does not receive the same treatment as a difference favoring the E group. The researcher in this case divides the calculated difference favoring the E group only by the total number of unique combinations.

IV. POWER

"There are only two possible decisions that can be made when testing a null hypothesis: the researcher can reject it as probably false or accept it as probably true. In each case, the decision can either be right or wrong, although the researcher can never be sure which. It is possible, however, to estimate how likely the decision to reject H_0 was to be incorrect by computing the significance level of the relationship, sometimes called the probability of Type I error, which of course implies the existence of a Type II error as well.

"Type II error occurs only when the researcher *fails* to reject H_0. In this case Type I error is completely irrelevant, but obviously error could be present just as easily in failing to find a significant relationship as in finding one. Just as obviously, the researcher will never know for sure whether the decision to accept H_0 as probably true is right or wrong, but again the likelihood of making such an error can be estimated although the process is more complex.

"At first glance, these two sources of error may appear to be independent of one another since only one genre need be considered for any one study (Type I error is irrelevant when failing to reject H_0; Type II irrelevant when succeeding in rejecting H_0). The two concepts are very closely related. The reason for this is probably best illustrated through the concept of power and its relationship to statistical significance.

"Power is defined as the probability of rejecting the null hypothesis when it should be rejected (that is, when in 'reality' it is false) and is really nothing more than 1 minus Type II error. Since statistical significance determines whether or not the null hypothesis is rejected, the same parameters that influence statistical significance also influence power (and hence Type II error). Power, then, like statistical significance, is a function of the alpha set by the researcher prior to the study (the more stringent the alpha, the lower the power), the homogeneity of the subjects (the more homogeneous the criterion scores within groups, the greater the power), the difference between the groups with respect to the dependent variable (the greater the difference between groups, the greater the power), and the relative size of the sample (the more subjects participating in a study, the greater the power)." (p. 27)

Appendix G

Product of the Inquiry:
The Research Report (Qualitative)

I. TYPES OF REPORTS

    A.   Case report of one person, event, or institution presenting a single picture of a phenomenon in its entirety or in various stages over time

    B.   Narrative composite report portraying findings pertaining to a group versus one individual

    C.   Critical incidents

    D.   A grounded theory

    E.   A cultural ethnography

    F.   A phenomenological description

    G.   A historical narrative

II. ELEMENTS OF THE REPORT

    A.   Problem or question

    B.   Detailed summary of the context/summary

    C.   Sample size and setting

    D.   Time and length of the inquiry

    E.   Researcher-participant relationship

    F.   Thorough representation of transactions

    G.   Detailed articulation of the methodology, including data gathering techniques, analytical procedures, investigator assumptions and biases, and procedures taken to ensure the rigor of the study

    H.   Comprehensive discussion of the results of the inquiry, interpretations supported with substantive evidence and examples from the data, findings compared and contrasted with existing literature and theoretical perspectives

Index

('i' indicates an illustration; 't' indicates a table)

131

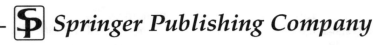 *Springer Publishing Company*

Encyclopedia of Nursing Research

Joyce J. Fitzpatrick, PhD, RN, FAAN

"This book is a must for any serious historian and researcher. The encyclopedia is an invaluable source for students of research, and researchers interested in outcome measures and the development of health policy."
—*Faye G. Abdellah,* EdD, ScD, RN, FAAN
Dean and Professor, USUHS Graduate School of Nursing

First of its kind! Written by the world's leading authorities in nursing research, ENCYCLOPEDIA OF NURSING RESEARCH highlights: over 200 contributors; over 300 articles; key terms and concepts in nursing research, and features an extensive cross-referenced index. Topics include: nursing services; nursing education; nursing care; specialties in nursing; patients' reactions and adjustments; nursing organizations and publications. Readily accessible to students and professionals, this volume is written for the information-seeking professional engaged in research issues and for those beginning their studies in nursing or related health research.

A Sampling of Entries:

- Advanced Practice Nursing
- Applied Research
- Clinical Nursing Research
- Computer-Based Documentation
- Family Caregiving to Frail Elderly
- Feminist Research Methodology
- Geriatrics
- Glossary of Acronyms
- Henderson's Model
- Internet
- Journals in Nursing Research
- Measurement and Scales
- Nursing Informatics

1998   752pp   0-8261-1170-X   hardcover

536 Broadway, New York, NY 10012-3955 • (212) 431-4370 • Fax (212) 941-7842